Praise for *Breaststrokes*
by Cathy Edgett and Jane Flint

"Through poetry, journaling, and reflecting back, Cathy and Jane intimately share with us their discovery and exploration of the movement and stillness that reside as powerful resources within each of us."

— **Karen Roeper, founder of Essential Motion**

"Reading this book, feelings surfaced in me, wishes that I had someone to go through the journey of my illness as Cathy had in Jane."

— **Charlotte Melleno, MFT**

"You would think that every observation, every reflection, would have been written by now about breast cancer. But this gift of a book—created by two bosom friends—shares both their fresh, accessible poetry, and the thoughtful entries of a meditative, hopeful, yet realistic blog. Read it to bolster your spirit. Or give it to someone who understands."

— **Karin ß. Miller, The Cancer Poetry Project**

"This compassionate diary of the abiding friendship between two woman during the illness of one, is without a doubt one of the most inspirational, honest, and beautifully written works I've ever read on the subject of breast cancer."

— **Patricia V. Davis, award-winning author of**
Harlot's Sauce

Harper Davis Publishing

Breast Strokes

*Two Friends Journal Through the
Unexpected Gifts of Cancer*

Cathy Edgett is a poet, writer, and a Rosen Method Bodywork Practitioner. She feels blessed to also be a treasured wife and mother. Her unique experience with cancer became a springboard for much of what she's learned about the human condition, and the incentive for this book. She enjoys her blog, *Heart Happy* (**http://cathy-edgett.livejournal.com**) and the connections it inspires.

Jane Flint has an extensive background in human development, health advocacy and communications. She also is a wife, mother, and lifelong writer. With Karen Roeper, she created "Eyes of the Beholder", a series of workshops leading participants into a greater awareness of themselves through the use of movement and video.

Cathy and Jane both live in the San Francisco Bay Area. Both continue to enjoy good health and peace, and remain the closest of friends.

To download Readers Guides for this book, and for more
information, visit: www.cathyandjane.com

This title is also available as an e-book

Breast Strokes

Two Friends Journal Through the
Unexpected Gifts of Cancer

By Cathy Edgett and Jane Flint

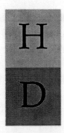

Harper Davis Publishers

Harper Davis Publishing, Inc.

Published in the United States of America by Harper Davis Publishing

Edgett, Cathy.
Breast strokes : two friends journal through the unexpected gifts of
cancer / Cathy Edgett, Jane Flint. -- 1st American pbk. ed. – La
Vergne, TN : Harper Davis Pub. Co., c2010.
p. ; cm.
ISBN: 978-0-9819153-9-5 (13 digit) ; 0-9819153-9-6 (10 digit)
1. Breast--Cancer--Patients--Biography. 2. Breast--Cancer--Patients--
Diaries. 3. Breast cancer patients' writings, American. 4. Female
friendship. I. Flint, Jane, 1948- II. Title.
RC280.B8 E34 2010 2009943519
362.196/994490092--dc22 1002

Printed in the United States of America
Set in Garamond, Georgia and Microsoft Sans Serif

Dedicated to my family, friends, community, and Cat Mandu.

- Cathy

Dedicated to the memory of Barbara Smith Didario and with many thanks to my husband, Jim Mayer, who supported Cathy's and my writing by making my breakfast every morning.

- Jane

Every moment is a moment.

Every moment has a certain request on us.

The question is how we answer it ...

Charlotte Selver — 1901-2003

Preface

Diagnosed with breast cancer, I made two decisions that augmented my nine month path through treatment. One was to take the advice of my older son and create a blog, an online, interactive journal that allowed accessibility and undemanding touch with family and friends. The other was to ask my friend Jane, with whom I had a writing relationship, to write with me each weekday morning at seven. Within two weeks after surgery, I had a blog called *Heart Happy,* which my friend Vicki called *Cathy's Heart,* and I was posting daily reports on my journey through cancer treatment. Each weekday I called Jane, and after speaking, we would hang up, and each write separately. Then she would call, and over the phone, we would each read what we had written. We delighted in shared ideas and images. Our writing time became meditation and medication for us both.

We learned about friendship, and discovered that in honoring the writing commitment, we were coming to know ourselves and each other in a more inclusive way. My medically imposed stillness rippled through Jane and out into the world. Edges blurred. Some mornings we had ten minutes and other mornings we had sixty, but each time we wrote, something new was revealed. We looked forward to our writing time, our date with the muse.

Poems became our outlet for what brewed within as we united in a vision for healing and health. I began to understand that I was graced to be part of a compassionate, innovative and responsible health care system. Robert Browning once said, "Grow old along with me. The best is yet to be," and so it has been for me.

This is a diary, taken from my blog. It is my journal of going through breast cancer treatment in 2005 and 2006 with the writing support of a friend, who was actively involved in earning a living and honoring her family life. As we wrote poems and posted them on the blog, we gave permission to others to write their own, and people began to share and post their poems, as well. My journal that had always been private was now public, like my body and my life. Through writing with Jane and through my blog, I felt purposeful, involved.

This book is my experience and interpretation, as well as Jane's. I understand chemotherapy for breast cancer has changed since I went through treatment, and it will continue to do so with medical advances. I am aware there may be a gap between what my doctors said and what I heard. I did not record my appointments as many wisely do, and yet, here is a record of my perceptions of what I traveled through.

My background is in the Somatic field. I am a Rosen Method bodywork practitioner and a long-time student of Sensory Awareness and Essential Motion. My intention throughout treatment was to use my skills, to pay attention and integrate my experience, to honor the natural intelligence of my being, and to not back away or try to escape by leaving my body or living in a huddled mental clench above my neck. I heard the voice of Charlotte Selver, my late teacher of Sensory Awareness, reminding me that my legs were for more than carrying around my head. When chemo dripped into my arm or the radiation machine pushed against my chest, I would repeat: "Every moment is a moment. Every moment can be cherished." In these nine months, I learned to understand the meaning of those words that had been illusive before treatment, to know that each moment, without judgment or comparison, is complete.

— Cathy

Connection

finds what gives
like the worm that enters through the autumn apple's bruise
tracks down the quirk that carries something useful
for the rest and holds what harmony can not.

Not even the apple hangs suspended in this world
without softening at the spot where it
leans into its being.

– Jane

Part 1:
October to December

Beginning: Cathy

For longer than I'm willing to admit, I noticed a dimpling in the upper-left portion of my left breast. But, my mother had recently died, and my book group was taking a trip to England, and nothing was going to interfere. With a full dose of denial and wishful thinking, I was sure a wand of positive thought would whisk it away. Finally, I went in for a mammogram which led to a sonogram and a biopsy. It was October, and I was fifty-five.

I was informed I had cancer in my breast. With a lumpectomy and radiation, the doctor said I should be done with treatment by Christmas. This seemed like good news, no big deal, a minor blip on my screen. During the lumpectomy, three sentinel lymph nodes would be removed from my underarm to ensure that the cancer had not spread beyond my breast. If they came up "clean" which "we" were sure they would, this experience would soon be over and all would return to normal, whatever that might be. I found it difficult to share the news because of how it affected others, so I parceled it out and told only a few friends each day.

My husband, Steve, and our two sons, Jeff, 31, and Chris, 28, were there for me in full support. I spent only one night in the hospital and went home to heal. I was told not to lift anything or type for two weeks. Since I am an email-addict, I typed through the pain.

Then, I received another call.

The post-operative biopsy showed cancer in my lymph nodes, and chemotherapy would now become part of the treatment to kill off any other cancer cells remaining in my body. I would lose my hair, and the overall treatment would last until late May or early June. Because of my "excellent" health, the doctor proposed "hard" chemo, which takes place every other week, rather than every third week. This way, I would finish chemo in four months rather than six.

People asked how it felt. My son was with me when the call came, and we sobbed together. Flowers were left at the door as we cried. Then, it was time to fight.

With that, I began to slow. I understood the fast-growing cells in me were going to be destroyed by chemotherapy, so I focused on what is slow to grow and lives a long time. I discovered kinship with lichen, bonsai, and redwood trees. Muir Woods became a second home, and I found refuge in ocean waves, running sand through my fingers, and holding and caressing a newly-found rock or stone. I looked up at the

1

Sleeping Maiden that is Mount Tam, and knew there I would find rest. My sons moved home temporarily to help with my care, while our twenty-one year-old Cat, Mandu, created a healing space, and family and friends circled and snuggled in to support. Steve was, as always, completion and heart. Steve, Jeff, and Chris offered to shave their heads in support, but, in my opinion, one bare head was enough. We were set to begin.

The Painting Life

I paint with "light portrait pink,"
rose, yellow, burgundy, and gold,
title the result,
"Meditation on Becoming Flesh",
then, "Healing Power of Flesh",
and conclude, "The Cradle of God".
I place the canvas on a chair
where the painting sits subdued
until a certain time in the late afternoon
when sunlight hits it through the window
and leaves
dance like bubbles
creating a space
for prophets
and monks
to speak.
I watch entranced
when shadows dance
aliveness on the skin
of what I made,
feeling inside the wind.

— Cathy

Beginning: Jane

When Cathy first told me about her diagnosis, I knew I wanted to help. Fifteen years earlier, I had lost my friend, Barbara, to breast cancer while she was still a young mother. I hadn't found a way to be with her during her illness, and I still felt sad about that. So even though Cathy lived forty miles away, and I had a full time job, a son in college, a mother in her mid-eighties, and a husband, Jim, with whom I very much enjoyed spending time, I didn't want to miss this chance to help. Somehow, I imagined, I could make the trip once in a while to do her shopping, make food, and maybe take her to appointments when Steve was out of town on business. Instead, she asked me to call her every weekday morning and write with her. Although we are both writers and had an on-again, off-again writing partnership for several years, I wondered how making such a commitment could be of use to her in her illness. Still, I agreed.

On our first morning of writing together, I was sitting in the busy foyer of an office building, waiting to attend a management training session for work. As Cathy and I spoke on the phone, people bustled all around me with their Blackberries and briefcases. They were all going somewhere. But I was sitting still, in the middle of it all, wondering, how could I be with my friend through this illness?

As I sat, the image of a bird building its nest appeared to me. At first, the place that became the center of the nest was undefined — just another part of the living, breathing world. As the bird placed its twigs, that point became more still, more dry, more sheltered. When we spoke by phone about what we each had written that morning, we found we'd both written about birds. Although I had written about the bird's still point as its place of shelter, and Cathy had written about the still point in the bird's breast from which flying emerges, we were both pleased with the synchronicity of our bird images. I felt a glimmer of hope that I could, with my words, create a place of safety for Cathy and feel connected to her in spite of the distance. Maybe this act of support could be simpler than I was making it.

After the first few weeks, though, my role began to feel very big. When I'd agreed to call and write every day, Cathy thought her treatments would be over in a couple of months. But then, her doctor recommended longer treatments. I began to wonder if I was equal to my commitment. I realized Cathy's needs could change every day, and I started to question what it meant to write together. Should I offer feedback and critique? Tune my writing focus to Cathy's? Make her laugh? Offer encouragement? Or was this commitment less about writing, and more about my presence and awareness, like tending a garden? If so, could I listen across the distance well enough to offer something useful?

4

Then, one morning, I began to sense that while Cathy's experiences were new, what we were doing together was familiar. Cathy was being a writer. On the one hand, like the best of writers, she never looked away from what was happening. She distilled detail and essence and shared it with anyone who read her blog. "Here's what the world looked like today," she would say, either from chemo, from radiation, or from wherever she was. On the other hand, she used the tools of a writer to create a story ahead of her, a story that often drew on both the natural world around her - Mt. Tamalpais, Muir Woods, the sea, or the seasons - and on her family life and celebrations; through these, she imagined life without or beyond illness. I also realized that day she was asking two things of me. One was to be a witness with her of the very real possibility of her death, and to meet that by reporting the experiences I felt in each moment. The other was to help her maintain contact with life outside of illness. As those requests sank into my awareness, a new question arose: "How will I be changed?"

Now, at the end of her cancer treatments, the nest I built for Cathy on that first day of writing means something different to me. Now I sense it wasn't Cathy who needed the nest's protection so much. It was me. Cathy needed to stay in touch with her vitality, with movement, and with the possibilities of the future. I needed a place to go that was sheltered from the busy outside world, a place where it was safe to really be alone with myself and with the feelings that come up when a friend walks close to the line between life and death. I needed a place where I would allow myself to feel life and death every day and speak to those feelings.

I began to see that even though I had been writing poems and stories since I was small, I'd rarely devoted time to myself to write before Cathy's illness. I certainly had never given myself time to write first thing in the morning, every morning, with the newest eyes of the day. I realized that by making time for Cathy, I had made room in my life for writing. More than that, I'd allowed myself time each day to really notice and inhabit my life, acknowledging that, like Cathy, I am "living while dying" each day, as the poet Stanley Kunitz said. Now, every day, when I make the time to write, I find moments that are imbued with the importance and beauty of the moment that, prior to Cathy's illness, I had not acknowledged regularly.

My instinct to give something to Cathy has transformed itself into this gift to myself.

The Gardener

Yesterday
he moved the lavender to a spot
closer to the sun
placed its roots into a well-drained soil
and in the damp place that it left
planted sage and thyme. He reassigned the blue grass
that had volunteered around the maple
into the bald spots on the lawn and in its place
planted hakone grass, pushed the root-bound
cylinder of dirt out of its nursery pot
and quartered it, the naked nerve-like tendrils
shy in light and raw. Some roots, some blades
were sacrificed. Even though he worked as quickly
as he could, brought the water to each one,
they all looked a little weary. Before he left
as night descended deep
he circled round and pressed each plant into
its new-found ground
unflinching, tender.

– Jane

Recovering From Surgery

October 26:

When I was feeling down this morning, my older son Jeff suggested I begin a blog, an online journal, and so I did. And, here I am. It seems a bit weird, but a blog is the modern way to go, and if I think of it as a way of staying in touch with family and friends, I see it is not egocentric or boring, but helpful, and maybe even tantalizing, scintillating, and riveting. I am beginning to understand that people are interested in my experience. Two weeks since the operation, two weeks, and now the sound of rain. I'm not supposed to type, but I do.

Pastured

> *Now I understand my mother*
>
> *wanting*
>
> *to do her own laundry,*
>
> *shop, and drive.*
>
> *I, too, hold to these tasks*
>
> *symbolizing freedom.*
>
> *For her, each letting go,*
>
> *was another stone removed*
>
> *from the fence*
>
> *that kept her here.*
>
> *She roams in mountains I cannot see.*

> *I will be well again.*
>
> *I am.*

— Cathy

October 27:

In the moment, I am on hold, and trying to integrate that my only purpose until I heal from the surgery is to rest and receive.

Pain has reined me in. It has taken me awhile to realize that when I bend over, I hurt, and so maybe I can ask someone to help me with my chores. I was viewing this as vacation time, so I was whizzing around to the beach and carrying logs in for the fireplace. Now I realize, with my adrenaline used up, I am worn out. I am learning to be and to accept I need time in order to recover from surgery. I begin to contemplate the words of Charlotte Selver, my teacher of Sensory Awareness: "This moment is the moment." Perhaps, each moment is an anchor, a place to rest.

The other day I sat in the car at Tennessee Valley. In the past, I've had a rather low opinion of people who drive to a beautiful spot and don't even get out of their car to walk around, but I had no energy to open the door, though I did push the button to whirl my window down. I was reminded of a little girl who thought hand-cranked windows were magical because they worked with the engine of the car turned off. Even though I was pushing a button rather than cranking, there was magic.

Suddenly, I was everyone I saw, the little girl taking horse-back riding lessons, the older couples changing out of their walking shoes into fancier ones, and the sleek young men on their bicycles. I was the group of high school cross-country runners and the person who stopped to use the port-a-potty. I shared their sweat, and felt centered in their swirl. I had been feeling like an old, useless bag, but now I saw myself as Santa's bag of presents, filled with gifts.

On the other hand, I never thought so much would be taken away so quickly. Reading is no longer a comfort, and walking is limited. My eyes increasingly fill with tears. Marion Rosen, founder of Rosen Method, says that "tears are liquid love." I bathe.

My totem has changed from the mountain lion to the chicken. I now have great respect for chickens, and expand to feel my fear as much as is possible at this time. My lesson is simply to be and in this being, I see how clearly I am you and you are me. We are in this together. I am not alone.

When Jane asked what she could do to help, I suggested writing. Today we write, and poetry is the form that emerges for us both. It seems right. Poetry is a way to say what can't be said any other way. Jane points out that with all I am going through, I am a still point around which others are revolving. I write of fatigue, acknowledging that I cling to life like the dry moss of fall. My well is deep, and I wade through stillness, an egret in a pond.

There are times when I think I will run away to Mexico and desert this medical regimen, and then something comes in to assure me I am well-supported in my stay. My mantra is "I am well." I don't need a mantra to know I am well-cared for. Jeff, my older son, doesn't need to work right now, so he, a man with a sensitive heart, who is also a chef of the highest order, is here to care for me. Each night he prepares a feast and we gather around the table. It is like when the 'children' were little. Steve and my younger son, Chris, also, sensitive males, fill in whenever they can, doing so around their busy work schedules. Jeff's fiancée, Jan, is here, too, as is Cat Mandu, who knows just when to step in and where. And now I have Jane and the blog. With the blog I connect to others, and when I write with Jane, I connect to myself. Connection is the key. I begin.

The Waiting Room

> *The still point*
>
> *where wings open*
>
> *and lift-off*
>
> *is still in the hum.*

— *Cathy*

Waiting Room

> *People criss-cross this space*
>
> *moving in and out*
>
> *they define my stillness with their movement*
>
> *like a bird lays sticks to make a nest.*

> *I am the one dot of unmoving color*
>
> *in the city blur*
>
> *My minutes move in a slow slur of time expanded*
>
> *against the rush of others.*

— *Jane*

October 28:

"The stars put down stems like straws from which to drink the sky." I wake to these words and Cat Mandu's need to eat and go outside.

Jeff has taken over the kitchen, something which I have been quite proprietary about in the past. This is symbolic. I'm letting go. The change began when I saw one of my many x-rays hanging in a hospital hallway for all to see. I was surprised to see the droop of my breast. They look okay to me when I look down from above. I stood there thinking this is how I really am. There is nothing to hide.

Carl Jung once wrote, "One does not become enlightened by imagining figures of light, but by making the darkness conscious." I peel off layers of hiding, and toss them like clothes I no longer need.

People now back away from sharing their pain with me. I assure them that pain is pain, and mine is no heavier or deeper than theirs. I am told chemotherapy will be like dying and coming back to life. I try to imagine what such a gift will bring. I envision myself as a rodeo snail with my hat tossed up into the air of the ring and coming down more slowly than I have ever known. A snail spreads mucous to cross razor blades. My emanations of connection will carry me through.

October 30:

Today I receive a forwarded email from a friend of Elaine Chan-Scherer, who has been diagnosed with a brain tumor and is preparing for brain surgery. Fascinated, I contact Elaine through email and learn she has a husband and two daughters. She asks, "What is a path of consciousness while going through illness? Is it possible to heal our spirits as well as our bodies?" Here are the words of Elaine Chan-Scherer as she prepares for brain surgery.

Dear Friends and Family,

Two nights ago, I woke up with great fear that I could die. Of course, I woke up Karl. We started talking and I really took it in that YOU are all going to die too. We are all going to die. I have the advantage here, because you have compassion for my possibly fatal condition, and so you give me all of this love. But we all need to be giving each other this love all of the time. It is only an illusion that those with illness need more attention. I can think of many people who are much, much more miserable than I am, and they are dying in their spirits. They need this great sea of love to surround them! You need this great sea of love to surround you!!! It is bliss.

October 31:

Though there is a painful reminder each time I forget I'm not supposed to lift a dish from the dishwasher, I feel great joy in receiving so much support to ensure I that live.

I've not yet met with the chemo oncologist, but I'm preparing; I read what I can, seek to understand. I remember fourth grade when I was chosen for the role of Rapunzel because of my long, blonde hair. Now, I let that long-haired identity go in exchange for life. I have a dream I am done with school and can now misbehave. In the dream, I am given a new currency.

In these last few weeks, I have gone from considering myself a solitary being, as I awaited news of the biopsy, to one carried aloft on prayers during and after surgery. I feel I'm on a journey to becoming a community as my formerly separate emails and private journal merge as one on the blog.

When I first learned of the cancer, I dreamt I was invaded by aliens. I understood horror movies and their appeal. Now, I see cancer as a chance to look closer at what goes on within, and then bring it outside to share. I'm on a date with the world.

This morning I wrote of the mole in our garden. His tossing up of soil and dirt, of what was previously hidden, represents the cancer now visible in me. Each day I look to see what he offers now, what he reflects of me.

In the solitude of illness, I welcome connection in all forms: animal, rock, and plant. I feel like the mole, forced, or perhaps invited to see in the dark. What's there? I am a rock, tumbling and polishing. What had been hidden is now exposed and smoothed. I am mole, insect, soil. I evolve, like art.

November 2:

I woke up this morning aware that my left arm was up over my head and there was no pain. I hadn't realized how often I sleep on my back with both arms up over my head. I love the openness of that posture, and that my left arm can now, again, reach up. I stayed in bed this morning feeling the beauty of the left side of my body, the feminine side. I've heard that for many women, breast cancer begins with the left breast. I wonder if we honor this feminine and receptive side of ourselves, the side so pumped with heart.

Today I go to the grocery store. There's pain as I lean to place each item in the cart. I request they bag lightly, and they in fact so carefully do that I'm surprised when I feel the weight of chicken breasts in one bag, grapes and bread in a second, and a carton of milk in a third.

Part of me is frustrated that I can't easily fill my refrigerator, and another part enjoys playing with the weight of objects as I move them through air. I am forced to be "all there" for what I do. Habit is gone. I use myself completely, and, with that, I know my vulnerability. I can't survive without the protection of my family, the community, the "herd."

I also notice that when I stay in the moment, all is wonderful. That is my practice now, this moment. I have no energy to judge or compare.

I open the blinds and light enters. This moment is full; it is enough. Charlotte used to speak of finding the balance, of never using more energy for a task than is needed, or less. I sense what is needed now. I have no energy to spare.

A Treatment Plan

November 3:

I shower through fear, and dress with care. My surgeon, Dr. Allison Smith, a total sweetheart who looks like a teenager, greets me with a warm hug. She explains that I am having problems because the incision cut through my lymph channels and the system is learning to re-route. Meanwhile, I am swollen and in pain. My very intelligent body will figure it out. To support my body in re-routing the movement of lymph, I envision trains all over the world switching tracks and airplanes changing course.

November 4:

My ten-year-old niece, Katy, sends me an email saying she loves me, and adds, "I'm glad that you're feeling good. I'm gonna ask Santa for you to be well. Think he has that kind of effect on people?"

The last time I saw Katy was in June. We were together to scatter the ashes of my mother. Katy and I built houses for the fairies. Katy says, "I live my life knowing that my Gramma, Betty B. Bartel, died happily."

November 5:

Such a flurry of thoughts, so much to share, and the first thought to share is no thought. Just sit in silence, alone, or with another. Look at trees and the sky, and breathe.

A meteor flashed across the sky last night, a giant match striking flint inside. I continue to cry easily. Time is melting and as I dissolve in that melt, I trust the world outside. I never wanted to take drugs, never wanted to interfere with this being I seem so smugly and snuggly to be. Now, I am concerned about this influx of chemo drugs. Will they change my perception of who I am? Who am I, anyway?

November 7:

Today, my son's fiancée, Jan, offers to cut off her beautiful, long, black hair and have it made into a wig for me if I choose chemo, which we feel sure I will do. She says she is taking better care of it than usual in preparation for giving it to me. I appreciate her generosity and know I can't take her hair. This is one gift I won't receive.

Until I Couldn't, for a While

I never realized how much I loved
the folding of sheets
until I couldn't, for a while
even though I don't really fold
that unruly fitted bottom sheet
just bunch it in a semblance
of a square, fluffy
like a park
with pockets
in the corners
like trees -

It is a closet jungle gym
for air to climb

Cases for pillows

the beginning

of dreams.

— Cathy

All my joys and sorrows hang on a line like laundry.

I am the line held at two points, one thread through time,
frayed and breaking, worn at an odd place in the middle,
repaired by tape
tied to a newer length of hemp somewhere else.

My ease and tensions are decided by the wind
its absence, presence pull on me
sometimes lightly
sometimes in heaving tugs and wild flappings.

You are the line in the neighbor yard
our lives laid parallel.

We are different but close enough to imagine being sisters.
From your yard you whisper to me about the moles and birds
about the laundry on your line
the bright colors and the sober privateness.

Like holding the ends of a jump rope
in a long ago school yard we swing our lines in double-dutch
over the heads, under the feet
of our children, our parents, our ancestors.

We sing out our fractures, our wholeness, our stories
our beginnings and endings.

– Jane

Looking Back: Cathy

During this time, I enjoyed everything and was grateful for everything, including the folding of sheets. I noticed folds and creases, and looked for air everywhere. Perhaps I was looking for spirit, breath, inspiration. I opened outward, fluffed like clothes when they are taken from the drawer, held open, treasured as they are worn. All felt so precious, each moment gold.

I was surprised to realize how much I wanted to live. Though my children are grown and I have had a good life, I reached for more, and in that, I began to understand "enough". I began to understand how much is needed for a task, to weigh the weight of what I did.

Jane and I were talking to each other through our poems, sharing stories, reviving the oral tradition as we read out loud to each other what we wrote. I felt supported, held.

One evening I stood at my front door receiving gifts of food, and Marlene handed me a hand-crafted metal icon that said, "Protect this woman." It did protect me, and I have since passed it on, and, in that moment of receiving, I felt a jolt. I understood how clearly giving and receiving are one. I loved to give, struggled to receive. Now, my heart was growing to receive all the gifts. It opened like a fan.

Looking Back: Jane

When Cathy wrote about folding sheets, I had no idea that something that simple could feel painful after surgery. It was meaningful and touching to me to be included in that awareness. After the first few weeks of being part of each others' daily lives, I was experiencing our friendship more wholly. I doubted I would ever again want to just "get through" a day, and my worry that merely speaking and writing together wouldn't be enough of a support, began to disappear. Sharing daily thoughts with another is connection. Without words, our experiences can slip silently under the continuous wave of life.

18

November 8:

My thoughts are with Elaine as she has brain surgery today. Jeff and I meet with the chemo oncologist, Dr. Jen Lucas, another beautiful woman who appears to be too young for the job. Now I begin to really understand that the cancer has metastasized. I am given a print-out of percentages and she emphasizes again that I have a choice in the decision, and gives me time to think. Jeff strongly feels that I have no choice, and that chemo is the way to go. The oncologist says to trust my gut. We aren't quite clear on what the percentages mean, and yet it seems each percentage point is everything. Though I fear the continuing loss of cognitive ability, I know I will fight for life. I can't take a chance that one cancer cell has spread and lodged in an organ, ready to create a home. I have a mole in the garden. I don't need one inside. Gut says chemo.

While I was being checked, Jeff sat in the waiting room and observed. He said he saw emotions close to the surface, like at a funeral. One young man came out of his appointment and was greeted by a group of friends who wanted to meet more friends of theirs at a near-by restaurant. He was briefly participating in the light-heartedness, when suddenly, just like that, something switched, and he exploded and bellowed that he didn't want to go to lunch. I was reminded of my response at my book group on Friday night. I was laughing when suddenly the easy assignment of planning the menu for our annual Christmas gathering seemed like more than I could do, and I broke into tears, like a vase of flowers tossed on the floor. I was awash in snot.

November 9:

The oncologist is right to make the decision mine. This way I commit to my own healing. She says my part in this, my attitude, is eighty-percent.

November 10:

Steve and I meet with the chemo nurse practitioner. Doing chemo for me is really about that small chance, that five percent that something could slip through radiation and medication. If I just do radiation, I am done by December. Do I choose to stretch this until June and lose my hair? I have until Monday to decide. If I choose chemo, I will start on November 21 at ten-thirty, when my surgery will have had more time to heal. Despite my trepidation, my gut is clear. I will do everything to live.

November 11:

My friend Joyce comes over to give me a guided imagery session. The idea is to help me find a guide or guides I can ask for advice and support when I need them. I see myself as a fawn curled up asleep among the roots of my favorite tree, a tree that overlooks the world, which is the sea at Stinson Beach. The tree is my guide.

November 13:

I notice that the tree outside the window where I'll receive chemotherapy has eleven leaves. Soon the tree and I will both be bare. I am also relieved to note that I can see Mt. Tam from the infusion chair. I know I can make it with the mountain as support. I live on one side of the mountain, in a valley at the foot, and now, I'll receive treatment on the other side. The top rises between.

Chris sweetly and enthusiastically offers to go with me to pick out a wig, which seems to me to be a daunting task. But after we distract ourselves with breakfast in one place, and lunch in another, it is easy and fun, and another preparatory "do" is checked off my list. I place the wig on the dresser over a crystal vase. When I wear it over my hair, I feel tented for termites. Perhaps I am.

November 15:

I read *Fighting Cancer from Within* by Martin Rossman, and I understand the power of guided imagery, which really is prayer. I work with my inner guide and healer, and go to sleep peacefully, and yet, when I wake, once again, there is fear, horror, terror. I cannot do this. I can't. How do I soothe now? Over thirty-percent of people feel nauseated even before they begin chemo. I understand. There is fear and there is nausea. Lance Armstrong said cancer humanized him, because it was humbling to be so scared.

I use the image of my niece Katy in her good witch Halloween costume to banish errant cancer cells. Her chunky shoes stomp on some and she wraps the others in the orange ribbons streaming from her coned black hat. They don't have a chance against the beauty of her smile.

November 16:

All these pronouncements on how we are changed by cancer — changed how, I wonder?

November 18:

This morning, my writing with Jane was interrupted. I bustled about instead of sitting to compose. When we spoke, she said she'd had difficulty getting through the door that she was trying to enter with her writing. Would it have been different if I had been holding my end of the thread?

Three Days til Chemo

I image myself as a swan

gliding along, feet smoothing back and forth

as I bend my long neck to feed.

Babies follow like habits I no longer need.

They grow and fly away and I'm alone

with the will to live and the desire to pump

my 24 cups of blood, 24 hours a day.

— Cathy

21

November 20:

We celebrate Thanksgiving today, the Sunday before, just in case. Jeff and Jan prepare a feast at their place. Tomorrow is chemo. Jeff will go with me the first time. I struggle to understand that it isn't an imposition, but a gift. This continues to be new territory, believing I give by receiving. 'Thanks-Giving' has new meaning. My family and friends are immune cells of support.

Night Before First Chemo

fear last night

feeling the play of musical chairs

wondering -

Is there a chair for me?

— Cathy

Chemotherapy Begins

November 21:

Today is my first chemotherapy treatment. This happens to other people, not to me, and I am here, or is it me?

Morning:

As Steve and I sit outside, watching the sun light the top of the hills, I work with the words, "I am not this body." I feel resistance to that, thinking, well, yes, but then, spirit flows through like the first fall rain. I am more than this body, but I am fond of it, too.

I want to be calm, and yet tests have shown that even before people are shown a violent or troubling image, their bodies are turbulent in response. Perhaps it's unrealistic to think that if I could be more present, more accepting, my legs would stop shaking. Perhaps presence is acknowledging and welcoming with kindness my shaking legs and nausea, the clarity of my fear. Can I find comfort in the energy of fear? Accept it as a friend?

Afternoon:

I got a big hug from Dr. Lucas just for showing up. She worried she hadn't "pushed" chemo enough. Her face fell, though when I told her of the rewards I have planted for myself to ease the way. She reiterates that this is hard chemo. It is every other week and there will be no good days, no place for reward.

I sit down and the mountain, my support, is there. I am shocked when the nurse sits by my side to hand-push the first drug of the day directly into my vein, because if it were to touch my skin, I would need a skin graft. I try not to think about what that means the drug is doing inside as it circulates and throws its weight upon my frightened heart. The next drug tears through my body like a flurry of wild cats. I want to cry, but when I agreed to treatment, I signed a form saying I would arrive with a smile on my face and would stay upbeat. Why, you say? Imagine it any other way. I struggle with tears as I continue to assure my heart it is strong and can survive. My heart and I agree; I will withstand and come back eight times.

I enjoy looking out the window at Mount Tam from my chemo chair. I see a hummingbird, fifteen flying geese, a seagull, and a turkey vulture. I don't read or play with the clay I brought. I enjoy the people and sink into the view.

Evening:

I don't think I've ever felt this bad. Perhaps I can't be as active as I had hoped. I feel spacey, and when I do gather the energy to think about doing something, I think some more and don't. A sun burns inside my swelling head. I know what it is to be a supernova.

I have medicine to help me sleep tonight, and tomorrow will be a whole new day. Steve, Jeff, and Chris are here, taking good care of me. True to form, I am able to eat. Jeff has prepared a delicious meal, and the four of us sit together as we used to do before the children grew up. It is like old times, almost.

November 22:

I wake and feel great, as though everything has washed through. Maybe I have a fast metabolism, so everything hit hard and then flushed out. I am drinking tons of fluids and intend to do the walking today, which is so crucial. I continue to see that when I stay in the moment, all is fine. Even during the worst of the treatment when I've honored my heart by thinking of all the support I am receiving, I've felt its answering tap, "I'm here."

In the afternoon I drive up to the Marin Cancer Institute for my shot to boost my white blood cell count, and that is when discomfort begins. Oh, my!

November 23:

I was raised with the power of positive thinking, mind over matter, and yet, this morning I sit and want to cry. I'm nauseated, so I drink some protein drink, hoping to keep it down. I'm trying to avoid the anti-nausea drugs, and deal with this as much as possible, on my own. Stoicism, anyone?

Despite the shot to boost my immune system, I'm so exhausted I slip into some odd sleep/non-sleep. Where am I? Who? I wake dizzy, sick, nauseated. I try to imagine what I am in nature. What is so depleted, and yet still lives? The salmon at the end of the run still lives, turning white as it rests on the side of the bank at Muir Woods, soon to be eaten, pecked, its insides exposed to sun. I feel myself burning up from within. Shall I lie here like the salmon waiting to decompose? Where is my will right now? I want to walk and step out, and I want to fall right back to nest, and awake as another me.

Being Human

The Dalai Lama chuckles
when we attempt to meditate
and instead fall into sleep.
The Gods look down

and know this being in a body is not so easy
like an egg being dipped in pain, like paint

over and over again.

Each level of dye

deepens the luster
until all colors

meet in the night-time sky

where after a time

stars weave through
and peer, like eyes.

— Cathy

November 24:

It has been a beautiful Thanksgiving. We enjoyed dinner at the Mountain Home Inn, which is part-way up Mount Tam, and overlooks Mill Valley and the San Francisco Bay. We were early enough to have a private dining room with a view and a fire. Nausea meant I kept one eye on the bathroom door. We returned home and made another fire from the wood from our dead apple tree. Lit, it blossoms out to a hollow core, and flames like a torch. I feel the same, opened, probed, explored.

First Thanksgiving Without My Mother

> *and yet I feel her here*
> *as clearly as the caw of the crow*
> *ocean eating the rind*
> *of wave*
> *clouds gathering together*
> *to cloak*
> *the sun,*
>
> *as it bathes –*

— Cathy

November 25:

I seem resistant to taking the anti-nausea medication, so here I am, awake in the middle of the night. I have woken to the sound of rain, and so I stay with the rockiness inside, the shifting that can't seem to find a place to balance and rest.

I feel earthy and tenderized, a log opened by fire and time. In the morning, I decide to imagine the aching in my head as the sun tapping from inside to open up the cranium, too small and tight to hold the changes going on within. Light is searching for new routes out of my head. This evening I want to light like a candle or sputter like a fire. No words. No need to speak. Jeff made yet another Thanksgiving feast. We realized we needed Thanksgiving foods shared in our home. It is a ritual of care.

November 26:

After an early morning walk, I am able to savor Thanksgiving leftovers. Nausea, in this moment, is gone.

My family gathers on the deck for the cutting of my hair. Everyone agrees it is best to cut it short before it falls out. I'm wrapped in our special pink hair-cutting sheet. It is a family tradition to cut our hair on the deck. Everyone loves my new "do." I see my eyes, and smile for the camera, pleased. Chris says I look "hip." I think of a phrase from Diane Arbus: "What's left after what isn't is taken away?"

November 27:

My head is burning again this morning. I am starting to get used to it and see it as a glow. The head weighs 14 pounds, or thereabouts. Today, mine feels like a giant sunflower perched on top of a slender, swaying reed. It is odd to me how an easy day like yesterday is followed by another like today. I stay with discomfort, and pause to rest the lids of my eyes, my head on its stem.

November 28:

Today I receive these words from a friend: "...when I start to write something that's a complaint, I censor myself because I think about what it would be like to hear a complaint if I were going through chemo."

We do not know how or why another suffers. There is no place for judgment around it, or perhaps, no place for judgment at all. And yet, this whole experience has me so aware of all the suffering around me. I notice people much worse off than I.

Sometimes I think the suffering of my family and friends is worse than mine, as I am in it, forced to be present, and I don't have much time or energy to think about it, to dwell, or perhaps, I am dwelling, but only in the moment. I only have energy for this, nothing more, and all I do is hailed as an accomplishment. I brushed my teeth. Hooray! I rose from bed. Clap! Clap!

My path is relatively easy. I am lifted in support, buoyed. I see how quickly life changes. There is pain, no-pain, nausea, not. There is so much shifting going on in me, and I have time to not only feel and write about it, but also to work with guides and imagery to move it through and understand all the images, feelings, sensations, energy, blocks, flow.

Today I make space in the closet for hats. I put away combs, brushes, hair dryer, curlers, and a curling iron I haven't used in years. This last object is such a clear noticing. Why is it taking up space in my closet when I haven't used it for years, and now intend to never use it again? I like my new short hair. I am a seal in the shower. Everything falls into place.

When the Dalai Lama was asked about the happiest moment in his life, he replied, "I think now!" Today I understand. This moment is all!

November 29:

I wake, feeling almost normal with only an odd ache in my head, like a boat rubbing against a dock without the padding of bumpers.

I thought I was well enough to face the shopping mall today. I was wrong. The noise, the bright, strident colors, and lack of true care were shocking to me. I've been living in a different world.

When I arrived home, I sent an email to those with whom I will share the holiday. I requested that when they think of going holiday shopping for me, they instead go out for a walk, or pause in nature, or just sit and reflect. I plan to do the same. At first, I thought that was enough, and it may be. But then, I also asked that they take note of special moments, and write them on a slip of paper. I have a glass bowl that was my grandmother's and I will fill that bowl with snippets of wonderful moments in this month of December, anonymous moments. Then, on Christmas Eve, we'll open the slips, rather than presents, and read them aloud. I do my part when I read an email from Petra that says, "Bald is sexy." I write her words on a piece of paper and put the paper in the bowl. Her words are a gift I want to open again and again.

I receive a group email from Elaine who had brain surgery on November 8th. She writes:

> *"... as I have said before, we are all going to die, and it would be great to live with open hearts without having to have a life-threatening illness. It would be great to ask for what you need without having a brain tumor! It would be great to receive love with gratitude and an open heart, instead of saying "no thanks, I can do it myself."*

I am shocked to hear that I will lose all my hair in 24 hours. I've held onto the option, or perhaps the illusion, of quitting chemo, but once my hair falls out, I figure I might as well follow chemo all the way through, even though thirty percent quit after they begin. After all, what could be more horrifying than losing one's hair? Now I sound insane. Today, I also learn that my white blood cell count is "very, very low." If it isn't up by Friday, I can't have chemo on Monday. I wanted an excellent report. I am a good girl, a good student, a great patient. I wanted white blood cells proliferating all over the place. I'm disappointed to have to once again admit that I'm mortal and need some help. I request that family and friends visualize white blood cells, and sit and think of everything that is clear, white, round, knobby, bouncy, friendly, helpful and conducive to my life and theirs.

November 30:

I've received creative replies to my request for white blood cell visualizations and I am now a boxer who leaps, bounces, jumps and jabs in response. I notice a change. I am patient. Well, yes, I am a patient, and I am patient. I can accept a delay in chemo treatment, because I no longer have the energy to muscle on through. There are no "shoulds," for how my journey is supposed to look. There is no fast route to completion, no record to break. All just is. The experience of chemo vibrates with the intensity and awareness of war. To live at more than a survival level means I play with the moments like taffy, stretching and folding them, over and over again.

Butterflies on my Socks

Why would I want to rush through chemo?

Isn't this moment giving me all I need

or could ever want?
Butterflies line up on my bright pink socks
like fighter pilots,

jets fueled and ready to fly.
Wings stretch down my legs and out to my toes.
They are, like burrs on my socks, going only where I
go.
We share good times, my feet
and the butterflies

on my socks.
I tuck my feet under the chair
and rub my toes

back and forth on the floor.

Tummy is content.

The butterflies on my socks

put the butterflies inside, to rest.

— Cathy

Lady bugs gather on damp stream banks.

Huddled together
they mass their small red bodies
like ripened seeds
on stemmy reeds and grasses
wait for the moment
when a chill wind moving east
blows by.

Then they will open
their polka-dot shells
extend their impossible wings
to rise and float on air
for days

and fed by the bit of sun
they've hoarded
from a summerful
of aphids

will arrive at the hurdle
of mountain spine
drop gently onto alpine soil

dream away
their winter.

– Jane

Looking Back: Cathy

My willingness to pause and be with the journey, instead of wishing or willing it away, was a huge step for me. This is where I began to understand Rilke's words from his Tenth Duino Elegy, where he encourages us to kneel and not "squander our hours of pain." Like Jane's ladybugs, I was allowed a place to drop and "dream away" a winter. I was nesting in the intimacy of our images, seeing Jane and myself as two wings merging in morning light. I was also aware of the support nature brings. I was held by the mountain, the redwood tree outside my window, the ridge across the valley and Redwood Creek.

Looking Back: Jane

Once chemo was inevitable and the rigor of cancer was clear, my commitment to this journey seemed to become very solemn. As the daily challenges got harder, I felt angry. I would have liked, or so I thought, to support Cathy in anger. But that wasn't where she was. Instead, Cathy's writing took on a quality during this time that seemed almost prayer-like to me, not prayer-like as in supplication or pleading, but prayer-like as Simone Weil and others have defined it: prayer as paying attention. Cathy brought to our time together a gentle allowing, one that she paid to each moment. It was an approach I mirrored and one that seemed to both slow time down and expand it. I began to see that for Cathy, being present right now was a state of survival, another way to breathe. In retrospect, it seems to me that by noticing all the details of her presence on earth in every moment, she imagined a way to stay here longer. For me, this intense wanting of one's own life was an astonishing idea.

Moving Inward

December 2:

I'm sobered by what's ahead. I've been able to drink coffee the last three days, and though it is a small thing, I realize how much I enjoy it. Three more days, and then, again, no more coffee for a while.

The truth of losing my hair is hitting more strongly as the days pass. I am attached to my new haircut, and having to let hair go again is hard.

Steve and I attend Cirque du Soleil as my last public outing for a while. Because of my lowered white blood cell count, I need to stay out of crowds. It is raining as we scurry into the tent for a night of magic and enchantment.

Winter Storm

No begin or end,

rain, creek, stream, pond, ocean bowl,

fish, earth, mammal, land.

— Cathy

Cirque

Of them all –

the spangled flier dangling from her ropes and swing
held only by the spotlight
or the silent clown who plays his common eccentricity
for our amusement
or the contortionist thin as straw
and the gymnast sinewed as a stallion –
it's the jugglers on the teeter board
that move me.

The group of them
in tune like insects, ants along a food trail,
fasten eyes and energies
in connection to the NOW–
Yes, we all agree, it's NOW–
and then fling their bodies into space

supernatural and real
as whales breeching

graceful without wings
serious
as angels.

– Jane

Three Days til my Second Chemo Treatment

Taste what is here now,
in the moist realm of tears held
waiting to fall and open outside
to slide down my nose,
and into my mouth,
a circular ride for fears
moving through like a line of cows in a field.

Bow to the taste
of the green of grass
one atom different,
than the flow of blood
cleansing the heart and lungs.

Adriamycin – Can I see it as cleanse?
red fluid pushed through my vein by a nurse
as I chew no-thought like a cow
pastured on the plains.

— Cathy

36

December 3:

I'm in the feeling of loss, that place where the leaf has said good-bye to the branch and is floating down towards the ground. Yesterday, I was looking up at the branch, wanting to thank it for all we've shared. Today, I am in the float, and one day, I will meet the ground. In this moment, I am here.

This morning I had another blood test, and I am confident the visualizations sent my white blood cells into swarm.

Second Chemotherapy

December 5:

Today is my second chemotherapy treatment. Though I have a cold, I am approved. Today was easier than last time. I went with a different attitude. I came from a place of surrender. I had no energy to fight or envision battles within. I was more relaxed and my heart wasn't racing. I knew it was fine to just sit, and so I did. Instead of rushing from one visualization to another, and worrying if I was spending the right amount of time on each, I just sat there feeling my organism as intelligent. I didn't need to direct, just trust. The trees have lost their leaves and the mountain stands, ease and comfort for my heart, eyes, and feet.

Mt Tam

I see you

and place my pain on your slopes.

You carry my pack.

You hold my hope.

— Cathy

Rainclean

The day rises in abundance

gladdening everything under its canopy

a celebration of small things:

morning moonrise

the cow whose nose

froths the grass

with pearled breaths

and dew and rain

one upon the other

free

for now

of sorrow.

– Jane

December 6:

So, just like that, to match the falling leaves of autumn, my hair falls softly into my hands in the shower. It falls sweetly, after growing so mightily right up to the end. I am proud of my hair follicles and their enthusiasm for sprouting. They will be back in four months after a good rest. I look forward to the soft curls to come, as I also enjoy letting go of what has been with me until now.

Today, I headed back up to 1350 S. Eliseo for my shot, and there in the waiting room was a friend from my sons' school days. She and I were called in for our shots at the same time. It is all rather public. You sit in a chair and lift your shirt, and in the needle slides. Walking out together, I asked her why she was there, and she whispered that she has had leukemia for seven years. Because she didn't lose her hair with the chemo, she felt she didn't have to tell anyone. I can't imagine going through this alone. I honor that her process is different from mine, and I'm grateful that I've wanted to share this and so many people have responded. E.M. Forster wrote, "Only connect!" It works for me. I feel I'm living in a connection well.

I used to think my thoughts should keep me well, and that if I was sick, I failed. Now, I live healed, no matter how I am. The word 'heal' derives from 'whole'. I am whole, healed.

December 7:

I wake, jubilant. The wild blueberries in my cereal gallop like stallions through canyons, as space in my brain creates new forms and ways to see.

I enter the shower stall singing. Then, there is shock. My hair, all of it, is coming out in clumps. This is no gentle fall. It gathers and clogs the drain. I thought I was prepared. I'm not. My head is cold.

Anguish slides through my fingers.
Silk gathers in the shower drain.

I lean down and pick up the clump, clumps,
pubic hair, too — and again

it is hard to absorb
softness leaving
softening to absorb even more
the love
surrounding me now —

I rain
inside
and out.

— Cathy

December 8:

The nursery rhyme rumbles forth: "Fuzzy Wuzzy wuz a bear. Fuzzy Wuzzy had no hair. Fuzzy Wuzzy wasn't fuzzy, wuz he?"

I count my toes this morning. I have ten toes, ten fingers, two legs, feet, and arms, complete with elbows, joints, and knees. Why then, am I sad? Why does the loss of hair pull me down? Hair means grooming, connection, identification, and yet without my hair, my eyes are huge. I am complimented on my looks more than ever before. I am given a permission I don't yet understand. People reach to touch me as though I am pregnant, with child, the child within.

I bought a new purse today, which motivated me to clean out the scraps of paper and notebooks that have accumulated in the depths of the last one. I'm surprised to discover, snuggled in the nest of my old purse, notes and thoughts from when my mother died. It is all here, those last few days of her releasing and my going back to Connecticut. Reading my words again, I feel her close, warmly and preciously close. Her white, laced handkerchief is there too. I hold it close, and then place her hanky in my new purse as support.

41

December 9:

I am awake in the night. I tried sleeping, but I've never slept in a hat before. It's not easy to sleep in a hat, and if I don't, I'm cold. In my hat, I look like an elf. Without my hat, I see my humanity. I feel androgynous, and not. I like my forehead. I have a strong forehead and strong shoulders. I am in molt, seeing my bones. This comes from Elaine today:

> *"When a goose gets sick, or is wounded by gunshots and falls out of formation, two other geese fall out with that goose and follow it down to lend help and protection. They stay with the fallen goose until it is able to fly, or until it dies. Only then do they launch out on their own, or with another formation to catch up with their group.*
>
> *I know that you feel the lift from all those people who are giving you love.?"*

December 10:

Cat Mandu is here with me, honoring my morning check-in with Jane. I am not feeling well these last few days, so I am resting. I lie in bed and look out, entranced with the beauty of my garden. Knowing when I am weak and need his help, Mandu places his warm, furry, purring body as close to me as he can. He snuggles on my heart and lap, watches the cursor march across the computer screen as I type. He is my friend, and one of my guides.

A dear friend of mine tells me she thinks I come across as "saintly" on the blog. I think what she perceives as saintly is fatigue. I don't have the energy to complain or do anything but surrender. It's not even two months since the surgery. I think I have been in shock these last few months; I may still be in shock. I'm not quite clear what's happened. I look in the mirror and don't know what to think. I don't think. I just look. My eyes are wide, absorbing. They seem huge to me, without the distracting maze of hair.

December 11:

I'm awake in the night. My head is so sensitive that it's difficult to find a way to rest on the pillow. Also, I have a cold and a cough. I decide at 1:30 that it's time to rise and uncover some purpose in my being awake. I see the stars alive in the sky. I have an email from Elaine. We are both awake, trying to decipher this world of discomfort, balanced with the glimpses of the divine from all the support we've received. I light a candle and share in the flickering waves. We email back and forth throughout the night.

December 12:

I woke up this morning remembering a sharing circle in Eyes of the Beholder, a workshop offering where I met Jane. Each person in the circle was saying how much they give. I remember being struck, as though with a stone, by the thought that this group couldn't be that unusual. With all this giving, who was receiving? Was giving being received, or falling back into a black hole to be absorbed and squashed, unused? I thought then, that perhaps it is easier to give and more challenging to receive.

Steve says how great I look every time he looks at me. I look in the mirror and see the head of a newborn rat. He says, "Cute Head!" I look and think, "What is he seeing? What is different about me?" I realize I'm happy. I'm really happy right now. I'm happily receiving. Each time I ask, I receive. I am "forced" to receive. This is my job. I'm showered with love and gifts. I'm grateful to receive, to shine like a sun, and to not allow what is given to sink, unappreciated, unclaimed.

December 13:

Someone sent me an article on possible alternatives to chemo. I read it and sent it out to others for evaluation. Once again, I came to the same conclusion. I want to live. Chemo may be primitive, even brutal, but it is what we have right now. I have to take advantage of what's available to me. I'm willing to risk this. I think when it comes right down to it, my desire to live is stronger than I ever realized. I made the right choice for myself. I wish I had words to describe how much I love being alive. Tears come to my eyes. Perhaps those are my words, warm wet tears, like the smack of rich kisses from the inside of my body to the outside.

Looking Back: Cathy

I was "in the moment," appreciative of life. I didn't have energy for anything other than breathing, receiving, and celebrating the simplicity of daily tasks. I remember trekking in Nepal where climbing was difficult, and awareness of the breath grounded each step. This was like that. I was the monk who carried the bag of barley to the top of the hill, and then collapsed aware, awake. I was grateful for my daily contact with Jane. Through her, I felt our writing explorations carried into the world.

Also, in looking at Mount Tam, I was pulled back to see the fullness of the breath, the rise, crest, and fall. I had hiked and biked up the mountain. I knew the trails, I knew where to push, and I knew where to rest. I was in a grotto, behind a waterfall, at rest.

Looking Back: Jane

Jane Hirschfield writes of proud flesh, the flesh that heals a wound and becomes a scar. As Cathy started writing about losing her hair, I began to think about some of my own scars. Each one carries its own stories with it: one from when I was washing dishes, one from the day I rode my bike up the hill behind our house, one from when I burned myself on the furnace in the basement. Each scar marks a moment that stands out from the many, many other moments in my life. Each one signifies a place of change. I wondered if I get a queasy feeling when I touch each scar because a bit of the sensation of injury, or perhaps even the event itself, still lives there. Cathy's words about her hair loss recalled this same sensation. I wanted to honor the top of her head, tender as a bud, as one of the places where she was being changed.

Compassion

December 14:

How can I not be pulled out of myself by the brightness of the winter stars and the colors of the trees? One tree in our yard is still losing leaves, and in the dusk the color is such that I feel kneaded like dough by the light.

December 15:

I woke this morning feeling tired of talking about myself on the blog. I thought, "Who cares?" But then, I honored the thirty minutes of writing time with Jane and the following words came:

> My wig feels comfortable. I'm at ease with it. It's not false. I am not my hair. Someone designed this wig, worked to mix colored strands so it would look natural. At a party last night, I noticed limp hands, and eyes that didn't see me. I was aware of those outside myself. Isn't that what this experience with the hair is allowing me? As I struggle with who I might be, I am still myself: an exciting, excited person, curious about the world and noticing others. I'm grateful I have a wig, yet I also don't need it. I like myself, both with and without the wig. Wearing a wig does not make me false. Nothing makes me false except when I denigrate myself, or say I am less than I am, or struggle to give myself thirty minutes to write. That is false. There is an ease to no hair. I have nothing to groom but my smile. I go into nature, my own nature, and visit the cells. There, Jane and I write and write and write. It is that kind of morning where winter light slowly churns, creams butter, warms words.

Winter Haiku

Dark and cold, today,

I move slowly, to, and with,

the kindling of light.

— Cathy

Winter Nourishment

oatmeal
dried cherries, cranberries,
raisins,
and cinnamon from Ceylon,
and now, a pink sky
after a setting moon.
An owl whoos,
too awakened
to sleep.
The sky
is one huge leaf.
We ride the veins
water and sap,
moving
inside
the creek and I,

do I

am I

feeling it enough,

the place where fire ignites

the in between

am I here for the dance of cells

the fairy springs

— *Cathy*

My surprise today is the love I taste for shadow.

I don't wish to hurry toward the light.
No longing draws me in spite of cold.
Its blue and purple, gray-brown sift
nestles against the lea side of the house,
my leg, the mulberry.
Quiet, not asking,
it offers deep forgiveness.

– Jane

Today, not quite solstice

As the last of autumn's leaves

answer the wind
with rattled throats
the sunrise has no color.
It stirs reluctantly beneath
its gray felt cover.
Before it realizes the
melted yellow
of butter in a bowl of winter oats,

I take a vow:

To witness the earth turn toward light and turn away each day
To drag a skate across time's frozen river and brake the glide
To catch the breath and hold it, let go slowly.

– Jane

Looking Back: Cathy

Because I was becoming more comfortable with myself, I relaxed and was more able to look outside and observe and enjoy; my self-consciousness dissolved. I looked directly at the world without the distraction of hair. There was nothing to groom but my smile, and I enjoyed doing that. I vowed to get my ears pierced when I was done, and I did. I read somewhere that piercings are invitations for spirit to enter. I figured spirit had been so busy with me, I would make an opening for it to exit when I was finished with treatment, so it could help others more in need than I anticipated myself being. Now, earrings flirt with the air at my newly-pierced ears.

Mount Tam is often called The Sleeping Maiden or The Sleeping Lady. She was a noble guide as I moved in winter light more deeply within. The cocoon was forming. There was time to wait for wings. I was in between like a log on fire. I wanted to feel what was happening, to honor each stage of my life.

Looking Back: Jane

For eight months Cathy and I took our breakfasts together. She sat in her house and I sat in mine, often with Jim bringing me toast and coffee so I could keep my promise to Cathy and to the writing. This commitment of talking, eating, sitting, making words in the freshness of a new day with the first energy that comes with sleep, is a kind of nourishment that has changed my body and life. It is something that before, I would have thought of as being "too much" to ask for.

Longing has been a suspect emotion for me. I've felt lucky to have what I've had, and some part of me has felt that wanting more of anything might "tempt the gods." But having this luxury of time, and hearing Cathy ask "Do I feel it enough?" during some very difficult times in treatment made me wonder: is longing the pure feeling of life? Is it longing that we let go of last? Did Cathy's longing towards feeling more somehow keep her here?

Third Chemotherapy

December 19:

Today was my third chemotherapy treatment. It was a rough day. I found out that the chemo effects are cumulative, so the chemo effects on the mind, as well as the nausea and fatigue, will increase. That was sobering. I can't imagine what I'll be like after this treatment and five more. This one really knocked me out.

Also, my red blood cell count is low. They did the treatment, but if it doesn't go back up, I'll be treated for anemia. I hope everyone isn't tired of helping me with visualizations. Red blood cells, Ho! Chemo world makes every attempt to cheer. There are poinsettias, menorahs, big smiles, and five boxes of chocolates. I don't want chocolate, but I do smile big. Then I come home and want to cry. I feel invaded, sad.

The medical staff continues to tell me I need to take better care of myself. Why is that so hard to do? I want to take care of others, to wrap them in blankets and serve them hot chocolate with mint marshmallows shaped like candy canes. What fun is it to sit here thinking about me and what I need? I want to give, yet my purpose right now is to believe I am here to receive.

When I walked into the chemo infusion room today, a woman was there with her husband and was crying. Slipping around her and into my chair, I learned from a nurse that she'll begin chemo in January. I remembered how shocked I was when I first saw the room. I wanted to reassure her that it isn't so bad, but then, I worried I would build up her hopes, because it is also not so good. I couldn't find an ethical balance for myself, so I sat quietly.

I knew that first day when I saw the mountain out the window that I could do it, that the mountain would be my guide and inspiration. It was a place I could internally climb, but today the mountain was covered in clouds. I knew it was there, but the crying woman probably did not. She could see neither it nor us through her tears. I have come to see that I am one of the lucky ones, one who is healthy enough to receive treatment. Chemotherapy is a diagnosis of strength.

I think people are changed by chemo because they have to expand; they have to imagine a world bigger than the one with right and wrong, and good and bad. Because we are healed with poison, we have to visualize what might be perceived as "bad" as good. We move out of duality into a wider space.

I had a lovely chair-mate today. He was so cute. He had shaved his head not knowing he would receive the kind of chemo where you don't lose your hair. His grandchildren think he's really hip with his shaved head, and now he has hair growing in where he hasn't had hair for twenty years. He said "We have to find the gold in this, don't we?" Yes, we do.

December 20:

I see now how the woman crying yesterday helped me access more of my own feelings around chemo treatment. I went in easily today for my shot. I know the routine, yet, though it may appear routine, it is not. I'm grateful the woman allowed me to see that this process is shocking, and I don't need to gloss over it, or say it is easier than it is. I didn't try to rescue her. That was new for me. I stayed with what I could do for myself. I looked within rather than reaching out to distract myself by trying to ease another's pain.

I am delighted with the rain, even as I simplify and wonder how far I can go before I don't exist. I wonder how many ways I can see each thing that happens to me. Is that what sun and water do when they form a rainbow to reveal the spectrum of light, and invite our eye to look for a pot of gold?

Morning After Third Chemo Treatment

I am this morning refreshed from understanding the woman who sobbed upon viewing the chemo infusion room. I am so used to it that I see humor, courage, and care in those who sit attached to a drip, many wearing bright, clever hats to hide a lack of hair.

I signed a form that I would be cheerful in my visits to chemo and yet I am not false when I smile, joke and connect. I prepare my mug of hot chocolate. I arrange my books of poetry and my talisman of the day. I read only a few words, words that knock deeply like croaking frogs upon my soul.

A nurse wraps a warm towel around my arm to bring the veins to the surface. With that touch, I enter tranquility. My eyes rest like butterfly wings on snow.

My veins flow deeply so it takes time for the nurse to find a way in. The first drip hangs like a vulture on its stand. The nurse hand presses the AC into my veins. Each time I worry and feel the burn. There are six of us today and three nurses. I sweep in and out of sleep. I want the vulture to know I live and yet my head bobs back and forth like a parakeet.

I feel anchored this morning. My angels have left their perch on my shoulders and are probing. I didn't know that angels are mechanics with tools tucked inside their wings. They pound and tweak every single micrometer of me.

I shake my shoulders and they peel, like wings, opening feathers to light and air.

— Cathy

Unmoored

I waken with a stiff neck

as if I have been straining

against some power all night

reining in a wild horse

or righting a small craft

in a storm.

The deluge has stopped for now.

The skies, still gray,

are scrubbed.

The clouds flap like the torn sheets

of defeated sailboats

even the mountain has run away.

On a day like this

how small

the calm center

on which I depend.

How steady.

– Jane

If you can sit and write today then so can I.

I'm not filled with an epic inner battle
or if I am I don't yet know it.
Except for the minor pains reminding me
I have one, I can ignore my body
so the old ways of work creep back in.

I get up early
not to greet the sun or stretch
with the yellow cat and Siamese
not so there is time to sit
with the minutes and the breath
as each one forms and fills and passes

So when the phone rang
and it was you

I was surprised, a little angry.
You reached out and pulled me up
through my confusion
eager for the air and words
like handing me a cup of coffee
piece of buttered toast
and saying this is your body
this is your life.
Remember.

— Jane

Two Days After Chemo — Each time, the hardest day

Though I set intention

to prance and play all day

two days after chemo,

energy is not ablaze.

Stop, I say! Halt, this rhyming haze!

Be gone, nausea, repetition, and malaise!

To bed, I head, to tunnel in my sleep.

Am I held together by aliens

who've never seen a human being?

I know my angels try, and I appreciate their deeds,

but I think my wings are hovering

down around my jeans.

Maybe I just need to sink into this shortest day

and make it even shorter

by wrapping waves in hay.

— Cathy

Looking Back: Cathy

Though at the time, I struggled with my feelings around the woman who cried when she saw the chemo infusion room, not wanting to view myself and my experience from outside, I have never returned to that room. When I graduated to radiation, I went to that building every weekday for seven weeks, and never once walked upstairs. Even when I return for check-ups, I do not walk the short distance to the infusion room.

Oddly, when I moved downstairs to radiation, I remembered chemo as comfortable. It shows how much we need to create the support of "home," no matter what that home may be.

I am also amazed that Jane was able to be so there for me, never letting me know that because she had a challenging job, it might be inconvenient, at times, to speak with me from seven to eight each day. She allowed me to feel I had a place in the world and that I was contributing, even as I dealt with ever-increasing pain. She gave me purpose, intention, commitment. Jane, too, meant home to me, and again, looking back, I see how much she helped to carry me through. Did I thank her? Not enough. That would have meant revealing to myself how much she meant to me. I wanted to believe I was letting go, simplifying. I don't believe I could let myself feel how dependent I was at this time. I had to self-empower and believe I was chugging along in a graceful movement, forming an arc of independence that was my own.

Looking Back: Jane

Even from the distance time has brought, it's hard for me to sit with the emotions of this period. I still recoil at Cathy's story of having the woman who saw her and others in chemo treatment, burst into tears in front of them. Even now I am surprised about the agreement each cancer patient made to enter chemo treatment with cheerfulness, so the experience could be tolerable for all. I understand why cheerfulness would be important, and yet I hadn't imagined the doctors and nurses would explicitly request such an agreement.

During this time the demands at work had increased. I found myself falling back into old patterns of waking up too early, thinking, planning, and worrying about work even in my dreams. Sometimes by Cathy's seven o'clock call, I had already been up a couple of hours and gotten lost in that place where work is all. After I had gotten immersed in work, it was very difficult to listen to the pain in Cathy's stories. Even after all the time that has elapsed since Cathy's illness, it's hard to read my words expressing both the discomfort and the irritation I felt when the phone rang one morning, and it was Cathy asking for our time together.

Young Light

December 22:

I wake before 5:00, meditate, and feel how stiff I've become. I'm barely breathing. I begin to move my neck, and then follow with my legs, arms, and torso; where I am led, I follow. I let myself feel that I have cancer that has metastasized. I have been avoiding the words, but today I realize that it's important to feel what's going on for me. I'm not this body, and yet I am in pain. My hands and feet are sore. Cuts don't heal. I have a cold that stays. The skin on my hands is too sensitive for light. I wear gloves for protection, warmth, a hug. My head is tender to heat and cold.

I went to Muir Woods today. I needed to know the salmon were there. Their return symbolizes rejuvenation, birth. For me, their presence means I will get well. The creek today was rushing brown with rapids. The rangers informed me the salmon are there, but I couldn't see them. They rest when the water is rough. My blood stream runs like these rapids when the chemo is pushed in, and I am given steroids. I understand why I am so tired on the third day and fourth days as I recover from the stress. I also have a revelation. I understand there is no core or any going deeper. There is only everything opening into everything else. I feel light.

When Steve and I went to communications therapy work with Mudita Nisker, I would say I wanted to go "deeper," and she would say, "There is no deeper." Today, I understand.

December 23:

I'm shocked at the bills for medical treatment. The numbers are unfathomable. Though I say I am charged, my insurance company is the one charged, and I am appalled. I also know my doctors are not getting rich. My care is expensive. Society deems my life worthwhile.

Today in the shower, when I notice the bones of my skull and face, I remember the words of Ralph Waldo Emerson: "This world is so beautiful that I can hardly believe it exists." I am comforted by the shape of my skull, even though, or perhaps because of the pain.

December 24:

Someone asks me why I'm resisting sleep. I believe there's so much intensity for life in me right now, such a desire to fully feel every moment, that I wait until I'm exhausted to go to bed. I think it's also why I wake up in the night. I want to explore every aspect of light and dark, within and without. I'm a glacier, calving. There is so much to know, explore, open, access. I don't want to miss anything. I want to be awake.

My grandmother's crystal bowl is filled with slips of paper that have magically appeared. We'll read them tonight during our gift opening time.

December 25:

Tears flowed when my family and I read the words from the Gratitude Bowl. I was stunned by what my loved ones wrote. In addition, we all bought gifts and shared the evening, deeply blessed.

My brother writes to say that my niece Katy rose Christmas morning and grabbed the glass from which Santa drank his milk. She wanted to get DNA off the glass and clone Santa. I savor this modern world, while questioning chemo, which poisons me so I can live. There are so many sides to gifts.

I never dreamed that I would lose my mother so quickly this year, and be dealing with all I'm dealing with. I smell my mother's scent in the house yesterday amidst the scent of the fire, the taste of the food, and the warmth of loving bodies moving quickly and easily to ensure my care. Full with the preciousness of life and its fragility, my tears keep falling. I am in discomfort, pain, and am concerned about what these chemicals are doing to me. I want to be here, and yet more wholly understand that despite all this, I won't be here forever. Tenderness is rubbing me raw. The petals of my being fall. Fruit forms underneath.

December 26:

I'm again awake in the night, a moon for the dark. My throat is sore. I look for something to get my mind off of my discomfort. I start to remember stories from my childhood. The Sugar-Plum Tree shakes goodies in my head.

When I go out to walk, I'm amazed at my weakness. I remind myself that suffering is only the desire for things to be different than they are.

I am resistant to returning to chemo. Being with my family shows me how weak I've become. When the caterpillar changes to a butterfly, its organs and tissues dissolve, creating a place for wings. I wonder if it hurts, if it is painful to transform. I can accept my discomfort when I view myself as a caterpillar dissolving to form my wings.

Jan was excited to go to the mall today and stock up on the half-price holiday paper and cards. In other years, I might have been there with her, but I realize I have no idea what will appeal to me next year, and I don't want to store extra stuff. Perhaps, most importantly, I now "get" that it is not certain I'll be here next year. And if I am, I can decide whether to shop. For now, I have enough, more than enough. My wealth manifests in knowing other people, in connecting through the heart.

December 27:

I feel well. The codeine from the cough syrup did the trick. I slept through the night. I still have a cold, but I am up and feeling perky, frisky. One odd side affect of chemo is the sensitivity of my nose. I smell everything. It's like being pregnant.

The five of us enjoyed breakfast out, and that was it for me. I came home to rest, just rest, too tired somehow to sleep, just needing to sit with Mandu on my lap, listening to two crows and the drops of rain. Jane says the lull between Christmas and New Years is a lullaby. I see it as accordion time; like a Slinky, it moves in and out. There are places to climb, rest, and fold. I slip into a fold and rest.

December 28:

The rain continues. The nurse from my insurance company checks in with me to see how I'm doing. Usually I say all is fine, considering what I am going through, but today, I say I am having a really hard time and am considering quitting. She is firm on how important continuation is, on how I have made a good start, and I need to finish it. I consider that as I rest my feet, which are sore for no reason that I can understand. The nurse assures me that Christmas is the hardest time, as we are out of our routine and the misery of treatment seems more obvious. Of course! That must be it. What else could it be?

December 30:

My intention for this New Year is to eat when I am hungry and sleep when I am tired. I am doing that already, by necessity, and I think it is important to proclaim. My peeling feet are melting and I can't wear shoes. My soles are earth. I wonder how many sunrises and sunsets open and close in me.

Interlude from Before

Rocks on the Beach at Tennessee Valley
The statues rise in the full moon,
A chord,
Stupas built to fall -

Rocks piled to stand,
like penguins,
looking out to sea,
an egg,
resting,
at their feet.

Each day the call
yearns to sweep the sea.

The lighthouse beam,

a beacon,
greeting the birth,
creating,
me

— Cathy

Solstice Time

Winter's angled day
has turned
the late tomatoes red
along the window sill.

The fan of leaf
whose veins
had caught the sun
has aged to russet.

Here in this stillness,
like the hand of dervish
at the center of his dance,
is knowing

the young light
will come again.

— Jane

Looking Back: Cathy

Jane was writing of young light, while I was playing with light like a baby in the womb. For me, all light was new and young. I was using light like building blocks, choosing what was mine to create.

I went back for a poem from "before," a poem about Tennessee Valley, a place where I resonate, though I couldn't walk there on chemo feet and fatigue. I didn't know Jane was writing of young light, but I reached back for the past, seeking the lighthouse as guide. Angeles Arrien writes that "Respect means the willingness to look back with care."

Looking Back: Jane

Winter was settling in. One day during our morning write, I started a poem whose ending spoke about the young light returning. When I read it to Cathy, her reaction felt larger than the actual idea I'd had when writing down those words. It seemed to me that she was attuning all her awareness to any feeling, idea, or thought that might serve the cause of healing. Like crops that align themselves towards the sun, she seemed to ally herself with words and visions that suggested vitality. She seemed to be providing her body with the visions and mechanics it needed; she pulled the covers up for it, letting it sleep while her voice told it a story of hope that would lead it back into life with the young light.

Part 2:
January to March

The New Year: Fourth Chemotherapy

January 1:

I wake full, happy, and grateful to greet and embrace the soft light of a new year. I look forward and back, honoring memories of the past and stoking intention for the future, even as I stand firm and fluid in this moment, the present. I am savoring my steps into this first tender sprout of the year, a sprout which will soon excitedly branch. Steve and I walk along the marsh this morning. It is still. My feet do well. I light two candles, meditate, and hang my new Reading Woman calendar on the wall. I go outside and pick a gardenia and a beautiful soft yellow rose named Peace. Flowers are blooming as I garden between storms. I come in and peruse the books that call to me at the moment. I am awake to pages turning and the soft whisperings of trees.

January 2:

I am again awake in the night, savoring the silence, sitting in subterranean exploration, imagining painting on an inner cave. Like our ancestors, I learn to honor the visionary state. The rain pours down and I visualize salmon swimming up Redwood Creek. Mandu is enjoying his new heated cat bed that at first he had rejected. He and I are both learning to accept technological advance, to welcome comfort a little more kindly, and to look for ways to warm and coddle our maturing bones.

I have been reading about shamans and their journeys, and I am struck by the parallels I find with chemotherapy. Understanding this as a shamanic journey, one which leads me to more strength and amps my healing capabilities, allows me to more gently greet the knocking down, and to more quickly seek the pop back up. Inspired by the words of the Dalai Lama, "My religion is kindness," I beckon a cauldron of kindness to simmer like soup within. The moon rises, a crescent of light.

January 3:

I am up, with a horrible cold and cough that I have been unable to shake. I so want this fourth chemo treatment today and to be halfway done. Steve is in London for work, so Jeff, Jan, and Chris have spent the night. I wake up, delightfully caved with my tribe. It is comforting to know there are warm bodies sleeping softly close by.

In spite of that, this morning did not begin well. Because my eyes were too red for my contact lenses, I wore glasses, which kept fogging up as I rushed around, and just as I was ready to call Jane, Mandu suddenly threw up. He did so under and behind my desk, past the vent, in a place that will be challenging to reach. "Grrrrr," I rumbled to Jane. "I am not going to write, "How do I love thee? Let me count the ways." I am going to write, "How lousy can one person feel? Let me count the ways."

As soon as I began to write, I thought of really lousy things, like concentration camps, prisons and burn wards, and I thought of how people get through it. I thought of what we always have as long as we live, and that is the breath. Of course, each breath right now is like shoveling a load of snow, rocks, and dirt. I am reminded of a poem I wrote for my mother, "Miniature Masterpiece," a poem about watching the precious fragility of each of her breaths as she lay in intensive care, knowing I might be seeing her last, as she did my first. Leaning into her breath, I gained an appreciation of my own.

At chemo world, I learned that next time I will start a new drug, Taxol, which comes from the Yew tree. That sounded friendly, until I read how it was discovered and understood that, again, we're talking murder. The good news is that there is no nausea with Taxol, though there will be tingling in my hands and feet. I'll receive Benadryl when I go in, so my body can better receive the drug, and since this treatment is five hours, I'll be dropped off, and most likely fall asleep.

I speak with the nurse practitioner about how rough these last two weeks have been. She says almost everyone has this cold and cough right now, and it's even tougher for me. Also, this is when the adrenaline wears off that has been carrying me through up to now, so physiologically, I am depleted, which affects my mood. It feels great to confide in her, knowing she understood. She works with this every day and knows how I feel. When my eyes filled with tears, she said, "We're both introverts, aren't we?" She told me it was hard for her to work every day with people, listening all the time. I understand. I understand why she does it, and I understand why I am sharing all this, something which might be perceived as private. There comes a time when we have no choice. It is the right thing to do, and we do it. We recognize we are part of community and connect. We take our place in the web.

Chris took me to chemo today and stayed, and we went out for lunch afterward and celebrated. I can make it through. My fourth chemo treatment is complete. I'm hoping Taxol goes easily. There is no way to know how it will affect me. What is happening with my feet is an unusual side-effect, and the problems will increase. So again, it will probably be no shoes or walking outside for at least a week after each time I receive treatment. But now, I am prepared. The air outside is sweet.

I remember the words of Eavan Boland: "If I defer the grief, I will diminish the gift."

January 5:

Jane and I speak in the morning, and afterwards, I receive an email from the nurse assigned to me by my insurance company saying she wants to hear my voice. I usually zip off an email and report I'm doing great. Today I call, and as we talk, I realize I am tired, just that, tired. I am fatigue itself.

Mandu curls up on the bed as a hint, and as I begin to give myself permission to go back to bed, energy comes in and I tackle my desk and bills. I renew my car registration online, again impressed with the modern world.

Mandu and I curl and uncurl new ways to view the world. Meanwhile, Jeff answers my emergency summons for help and arrives.

I realize that part of my quandary is trying to rest and be, while also 'trying not to try'. If I sit sluggish and not stimulated, do I go deeper within, like a mouse digested by a snake, or do I sit on the surface, an indulgent mass of flab? I think of cushions with feathers and touch my ribs.

Weary

"Poetry is the natural prayer of the human soul." Rilke

I open the blind slowly,
* unwillingly,*
wanting to stay in my dark place,
though now I attempt to ripen,
like the pink of the sky
* willing to rise*
* and open my eyes*
* and yet there is that place*
*   in me today of death.*

I consider placement in the sky in Tibet
*   torn apart and eaten this sore flesh.*
I am worn out, in need of a cave, achy with pain.

I need to lie down, let all pour out, release
*   all I no longer need holding me down.*
*   Today, I want to be air - no ground.*

— Cathy

Worry Prayer

One for Ira—deep comfort
One for Ann—freedom from pain
One for Jesse—awakening
One for Sally —days of play
One for Cathy —the long view
One for Jacob—a bright future
One for Persis—lessening grief
One for Susan—indulgence
One for Jake—true love
One for Lloyd—blessings
One for Gerry—sinking in
One for Janet—courage
One for Vicki—blue planet
One for Karen—forgiveness
One for Suzanne—contentment
One for Richard—connection
One for Shirley—love
One for Cecile—confidence
One for Martha -- endurance
One for Josh—a dream come true
One for Michael—softening
One for Diane—dancing hand
One for Peter—music
One for Terry—family
One for Jim—love forever

– Jane

January 6:

Instead of pushing nausea away, I decide to welcome it as a friend. "Sit here with me. What do you need? Some ginger ale, perhaps?"

Yesterday I enjoyed the winter sun, and I received a notice for jury duty. I do not want to call to request the form that gives me a medical excuse. I assure myself that I am young, healthy, and at my peak. I want to be part of my community. I try to imagine a scenario where I could do jury duty and I know it is impossible, and so I sit feeling excluded and banned from society. I make the call for the form. I take the excuse.

I have always thought I would like a mural on my garage door, and today, as I drive down into my driveway, the sun is shining through the trees in such a way that the shadow of the huge trunk of the pine tree is lit on the door, along with slender branches of plum. It's a delicate painting, like a poem or haiku. It's what I am right now, shadow visible when the sun is right, just a few syllables to summarize my whole.

January 7:

I struggle today with the unpleasantness of the chemo. I want to sit and cry, and sometimes I do, but there are so many hours, so many minutes, and I have so much time. The tender lining of my stomach says, "I've had enough. Please stop."

Presence

Today I don't see the mountain lion
only bones of deer
A rib cage fluent in two parts - a skull
hollow
as the space between stars
I see only footprints,
but, still, I ingest,
the exchange of energy,
the cache at rest.

— Cathy

Looking Back: Cathy

Jane and I began the year as we ended it, with writing our poems. Viewing chemotherapy as a shamanic journey allowed me to pop back up each time I was knocked down. I was weary though, and was looking for ways to part the light and sit inside. Energy was a continually beckoned and much-needed guest.

One time when I was with my three-year-old friend Zach, he was an airplane. He spread his arms and flew over a speed bump that was painted white and said, "Look at that cloud." I too, was creating a landscape, navigating a most unusual flight, where I could wing and make a speed bump a cloud.

The universe had given me a task. Ask and receive. I knew support was there.

Looking Back: Jane

By the start of the New Year, Cathy had made it through two and a half months of discovery, surgery, and a decision to begin the course of chemotherapy. Through that time, she'd kept her spirits up and also kept up the spirits of everyone who'd read her blog and daily poems. I too, had been enjoying my hour of being with her each morning and writing.

Then the day came that the weariness caught up to her. She announced it with the words, "all I no longer need is holding me down." I felt a kind of loosening, a relaxing of certain muscles, as if I had been holding my breath to keep this moment from arriving. It was also the moment I began to feel my own fear and sadness. I realized I couldn't continue to offer support to Cathy by simply holding on. And I realized I could no longer put on my public face at the end of our call and go out into a world that doesn't speak much about the reality of death.

I needed to offer a different kind of support: I needed to acknowledge the real possibility of death, not just hers, but mine.

I needed to recognize the reality of death each morning at breakfast, to feel the place that death holds in our lives. I needed to speak with her about my fears and worries. I needed to voice the hopes I have for myself and those I love before I die.

Tender Light

January 7:

Today I realized how much I need the darkness over the light. I am the mouse, swallowed whole by the snake, dissolving as I am digested, assimilated into a new way of time.

I am the snake. Every muscle and rib strokes the earth as I curve slowly, flip a tail, perhaps shake a rattle, adapt. I go to Muir Woods to look for the salmon. There are only a few. Both the stream and I are depleted this year, missing the inner stroke of the salmon's upstream fight to breed.

January 8:

I wake to the sound of soft rain and the realization that each of us is a star, a furnace blazing inside. We radiate rays of light, connect. I wake without nausea. Then I realize that though there is no pain, I still can't drink coffee or eat breakfast, so I sip chocolate milk and Ginger Ale. Steve and I set out for a walk and I am weak, so I surrender to limitation, return home, and enjoy what the day brings.

January 10:

Water tastes good today. I honor the change. This morning Jane and I speak of bowls and containers as the "waiting moment." She says I sound different, and I feel different. I buy a bowl, hand-crafted, the color of cream. I leave it empty to sit on the counter as womb or nest, full in its emptiness, open and waiting, just like me. I sense evolution, a climbing from the water, a place to be born.

Fog this morning outside my bowl which broke today,

> *so I could climb to shore*
> *where the taste of water refreshes my throat,*
> *and my legs begin to form.*

— *Cathy*

In the before, the world turned to face the sun, as today.

As today, in the after, the world will turn away.
Here in the in-between everything is itself, exact and true.
Again I wash the bowl that has waited on the shelf.
Now it has held my breakfast and will wait again.
It is not perfect or enlightened.
But each day it fills me with love and love and love.

- Jane

January 11:

My neighbor Mary dropped by yesterday with pink tulips and a pink breast cancer watch. She is bringing soup today. When we moved here, Jeff was just four, and Chris was not yet one. She was pregnant. Over the years, we've both been busy, and often seen each other only in passing. An intimate conversation between us occurs only a few times a year. Now, because we're both dealing with health issues, we meet to walk slowly and talk. We speak of all the strollers we see, the young mothers and fathers. It's hard to believe so much time has passed. We're now the age of those we thought "old" when we moved here. I wonder how many of us live, seemingly independently through our younger years, when all along we're intertwined.

Though I don't want to return to chemo, I continue to advise others to do it if their doctor recommends it. Perhaps, this is the division in which we all live. Life is not black and white. We have to discern and choose a path through the grays.

January 14:

Jeff calls, concerned that I've posted so little on my blog the last few days. I tell him I am resting, surrendering, renewing, recuperating from the last chemo regimen, and preparing for the next one. We lit candles last night and enjoyed a fire. I hum a creation of my own, "Sweet Lazy Days of Winter." I feel happy and soothed. My pacing may be slow, but it is right for me.

74

I loved the morning elimination ritual when I was in the Everest region of the mountains of Nepal. Each person slipped quietly away. I always squatted with a view. Why should my daily interview with my porcelain friend be any less enchanting? I notice what I do.

January 15:

I am contemplative, trying to better understand and feel into myself, to not run away, to stay somewhat objective, to stand back and witness. I am trying to balance as I look out on a day still uncolored, uncooked, just shadow, shade, and gray. Each leaf and needle is distinct, like fairy brushes waiting in their quest to paint the sky. The birds are ecstatic in flight and song.

We lost electrical power last night. I was listening to poetry, Billy Collins, and then suddenly, I was sitting in candlelight. Then the power returned, and then, it went out again. It was a chance to see which way I like it — on or off. I like it both ways, on and off.

January 16:

Today, I say it. I am depleted, tired, and worn out. I am scared. I am tired of having no hair. Perhaps this is surrender. Perhaps, I need to feel this more. Steve said his perception of the poem I wrote this morning was that it was in my head, not in my body. I am avoiding being in my body. Why would I want to feel how poorly I feel? I'm afraid I am of this new chemo regimen. I'm curled up inside against it. Perhaps I will spend today just feeling how I feel, acknowledging and beckoning my fear, and see what comes from that. I hear my loyal supporters pointing out I am fifty percent done, and I know the toll this has taken. Even my eyes are tired. I don't have the energy to smile, yet I know I will again lift from the mat and fight. The image that keeps returning is of crawling out of the sea onto land, feeling arms and legs form, and that first hefty lift from the ground.

Now it is evening. I am calm, steady, present, and clear. I see how speaking what is there clears the screen. I am an Etch-a-Sketch™ shaken fresh.

The old landlord was sick the day the rain began.

    By the third day water had flooded the clock factory.

    It rose up through the floor.

    It seeped through the doors.

    By the fifth day the water receded.

    The old landlord rose up out of his sick bed.

    He went to the clock factory and assessed the damage.

    He sat at his desk, wrote checks for the needed repairs.

    Everything you need to know about the landlord is here.

– Jane

Fifth Chemotherapy

January 17:

Today is the fifth chemotherapy treatment day, and I wake up aware that the schedule is well-planned. I am back on my feet and ready to be blasted again. Hard chemo, here I am! The nurse practitioner speaks to me for a long time before she signs off on letting me have the chemo. I am anemic, and my numbers are low. We talk about fatigue and how I feel excluded and sad, unable to participate fully in the society in which I live. I tell her how much I am changing with this, how I'm learning to rest and take breaks. She's amazed at how much I am using this to learn. She says others rail against it. Well, we each have our way, but I figure I'm in it, or I'm not. That's my feeling of the moment, anyway. She finally signed me off, because she said I "look good," even if I don't feel it. Taxol will have different side effects. It's a good sign I made it through the drip. My temperature and blood pressure were taken every fifteen minutes to ensure I was doing okay. I'll ache in muscles and bones, and have numbness and tingling in hands and feet.

We also spoke about radiation. "Radiation is not negotiable," she said. "It is either that, or a mastectomy." Radiation sounds great. She said radiation is a nurturing environment, very different from chemo world. I'm "ordered" to get massages. They are free.

The nurse closed a valve trying to get the needle in. An inch-high lump of blood formed in my hand. For chemo, they need a four inch straight shoot for the needle into the vein. This is not easy to do. I realize how little I know of the geography inside. My hand and lower arm are sore. I picture the veins and stroll within, trying to acquaint where attention has rarely been.

A friend tells me she was thinking of me and then heard wild geese honking overhead. She sees it as a sign of connection. She sees signs of me in the sky as I look for geese within. The architect Louis Kahn said, "The sun never knew how wonderful it was, until it fell on the wall of a building." I feel the same about chemo.

A paladin stands at your door.

No further harm can pass.

You waken to easy laughter.

Godlings keep your shoulders.

There is nothing that needs to be fixed.

Even the irreparable is fluent now.

– Jane

January 18:

When I returned to chemo world for my shot today, I decided to participate in an art class for cancer patients. I was the only one there, so Barbara set me up with a table-sized piece of paper, water colors, water, an array of beautiful brushes, and watched me paint. My abstract became a painting of me. My arms were long and reaching out, and I was well-grounded. I was on the diagonal, and I gave myself a huge heart that spread into wings. For warmth, I wrapped scarves around myself, and painted myself with and without hair. When the therapist pointed out I had painted over my arms, she said to notice when I covered myself up, and so I stopped and noticed, and in that recognition of when I covered myself up, I breathed more deeply. I don't need to cover myself up or hide. There is room for me.

I struggle with the indulgence of this, and am trying to learn to receive it. It seems odd to be sitting in the middle of the day with one person watching me paint. There is so much offered for those with breast cancer in Marin County. Diane Brandon, a Cancer Resource Specialist, told me that she went to Esalen for a workshop on recovery from breast cancer. They began by asking the women about their anger at their doctors. None of those who went through Marin Cancer Care had anger about their care. How could we? Our doctors are lovely, present and aware. We are offered free art classes, hypnotherapy, massage, counseling, and I don't even know what else. I couldn't do it all if I were well. It's a challenge to pick and choose when I am not.

January 19:

When I wake, I tell Steve the side-effects of Taxol are different than those of A.C. I feel terrible in whole new ways. Steve said I should write a poem like Wallace Steven's "Thirteen Ways of Looking at a Blackbird," only instead title it, "Thirteen Ways to Feel Like Crap." I thought "Thirteen Ways of Chemo Pain" might be more like me. I am in pain when Jane and I speak. I try to write, and then I go online and read about Carl Jung and the three stages of alchemy. When she calls me back to share what she wrote, we see that we each touched on alchemy. She began with the pain she heard in my voice. I, too, began with pain.

I'm trying to hold my right shoulder down

even though it keeps popping up to protect me

from the next blow.

The side effects of Taxol are different
than those of AC.
I feel lousy in whole new ways
like acid has been poured down my throat
and eaten out my insides.
I feel like a toilet bowl
where the squeaks of cleanliness
are squeals of pain,
and my hands and feet are burned
and charred.

I am taken apart, to understand of what I am composed.

— Cathy

There is a place broad enough to hold all pain.

There we sleep like spoons against our shadows.

Even at night under the moonlight we are safe.

We feed the hyenas and hawks by hand.

We become our true bright selves.

— Jane

January 19:

In the evening, I ask myself if I am well or sick. Then I realize it doesn't matter. What matters is how I am in the moment. Like the Velveteen Rabbit, I am loved even though I have no fur. Steve wants to take me to dinner, so I freshen up and put on a dressy sweater, a necklace strand, and my wig. My life is rich.

January 20:

Softness this morning as I sit and absorb what Jane and I share. She says it is my job to write how I feel, and I continue to come to understand how important it is to know what we feel. We choose the word "hop" to begin our writing, and I flow as she probes with form.

January 21:

I am again awake in the night, listening to the rain. My discomfort is extreme. I don't even know how to describe it, which is why I realize the doctors can't describe it either. I bend inward, like Kokopeli playing a flute. In this moment, I can't imagine recommending chemo to anyone. Maybe if their life were in danger, but how does one know? Bodies change. Lives change. Tumors go away. It has happened, spontaneous remission, unexplained by science.

I try to use the sound of the rain to calm myself, but this sensation with my legs and bones is hard to ignore. I try to imagine good things going on, my body firing back at invaders, but living as a battlefield is not much fun. I can't seem to find a way to relax, to accept, to find purpose in what is going on. I know this is only a moment, but it has been a long one, several days now. I imagine people worse off than I and still I can't sleep, and so it is. I'm awake in the night, enjoying the rain, knowing that suffering is to want things to be different than they are. Jon Carroll's granddaughter says to make our minds "ripplier." I imagine the rain becoming ripplier so it has more time to play before it hits the ground.

January 22:

Last night, I experienced deep, painful spasms up and down my spine. I went to bed early and slept for eleven hours, with Mandu resting happily on my chest. Now, after sleep, my lower back is tender, but not too bad. Steve and I walk out to breakfast, appreciative of each step and of the strength we gain in slowing down to see.

January 23:

I wake, feeling whole. I see the moon in the sky, hang by my arms from the light and kick my feet. I have nothing to pay back. I just am. I feel my place in the stars. While driving to my free massage (thanks to enthusiastic Marin fundraising), I realize how hard people in the medical profession are working to save my life. I appreciate the temple I am, the temples we are.

I walk along the creek and see coots, geese, ducks, and gulls, and a Buddha statue under a tree with a Winnie the Pooh bear dangling from the tree above. Life is like that, reverent, sacred and playful all at the same time. I'm grateful for life.

Today My Palette

I look for a vase
For flowers that come
Flowers I choose to pick

I am one in a network of stars
Holding my place
In gravitational space

With the curve of a smile
A bubble, I bounce, buoyant and clear.

— Cathy

January 24:

Today I consider hair. At first, I suffered at having no hair, and now I am happy to toss a hat on my head, content with that as grooming for the day. I don't even need a purse. Of course, I have the option of a wig, but what I observe is that people still like me and find me attractive, and maybe even more interesting and exotic without my hair. Plus, I can see and hear better without hair blocking my eyes and my ears. I read of children going through chemotherapy. They sound upbeat. I let myself be like a child.

January 25:

I wake, feeling a deep connection to source, like a leaf must feel from a tree. I see why petals curve and hills roll. Waves are flowing through me. Today, in my writing with Jane, I find myself writing of a mottled sky of blue and pink and the changing of the tides. I feel the in between, the place of transition and pause.

I have a nosebleed, my first ever. It may be the chemo or the dryness of the air. I feel well, and also sad. There is no story to the sadness. I think today I might touch the tears that I've held glacially for a while. Perhaps, the warmth of yesterday allowed a thaw, and I am feeling wholeness, the place of deepest feeling, the home of joy and sorrow.

After the dinner party, we went to bed.

We'd washed the dishes and silver, left the wine glasses.

Remnants of communion settled onto the table top.

The night house shimmered in the fissured moonlight.

From the places lips had met glasses a new verity was born.

– Jane

Guided / guiding

January 26:

I had lunch with a dear friend, the one who suggested I was sounding a bit saintly on my blog. As we talked, I realized that what I am really choosing to do is to fully feel this experience in my body. I don't distract myself when I go to chemo. I take a book of poems that will stimulate my senses, in order to more directly and evenly feel the flow of the chemo into my veins, the flow of what I view: the mountain, the hill, the tree, the birds, a sky that sustains. I am using this experience to more clearly know and honor the experiences of my body. I am beginning to eat when I'm hungry and rest when I'm tired. My chrysalis thins and builds over and over again.

Change

Vicki moves to New Mexico
Louise from New York to Mendocino
My insides shift coast to coast
and north to south -

Like a martini,
I am well-shaken –

Where will I come and go,
    frolic and rest,
      now that awareness
        of death
        grants liberty
          to chest, heart, breath -

The day turns slow cartwheels in me,

crossing the grass,

pebbles, rocks – I am guide, guided

to somersault on breath.

Are we trained to guide the path of the sun?

Mandu comes to be my muse,

A gentle fuse -

The cauldron stirs, stirred.

— Cathy

Once the danger had passed, tears.

She sat with all that had happened.
She lay her sorrows around her.
Not just her own, but any that surfaced.
They spread around her like a quilt
Her eyes filled its folds with rivers, tributaries.
Emptied, she stood there at the edge of endlessness.
Still it was better to sleep on the floor, away from windows.

– Jane

January 27:

I gather flowers in body and mind, feel them as emotions. The tides breathe in and out. Fragrance, like a brush, soothes. The breath is floral, violets, rose, and thyme.

When I woke, it was raining, and the stars were out, lighting the clouds. Now, the clouds blush pink, excited as octopi, in being seen in the playful exchange of inked night for day.

One

Mind plays golf this morning

Full swings shooting balls to the stars.

I want my touch to wing an exchange

Landing holes in one.

— Cathy

Turtle Light

Rain tinsels in me

Dripping shines, reflects

Light flashes on and off,

The stars gone,

The neck.

— Cathy

Honey Spot

Bubbling cartwheels in my heart today.

Exuberance sprays like gardenia scent

Thick enough to stand on

And draw angels in the sky to circle me.

I am hive.

— Cathy

Looking Back: Cathy

In this time, I often felt like Persephone, living underground, knowing I would rise in spring. There was joy in the depths, and exuberance and bubbling amidst the pain. At this time, Jane and I often spoke only a few words. We listened to the breath, for what might ride it unsaid.

I continued my intention to stay conscious and awake as I went through this process. I didn't read much, but what I did read was stimulating. I talked to Diane Brandon, the Cancer Resource Specialist at the Marin Cancer Institute and a breast cancer survivor, and she asked how anyone could read fiction while going through this. "This is it," she said. "Nothing compares."

I asked for prayers, and each time they came. The support was there, and my imagination threaded words into games.

Looking Back: Jane

One day in January, I wrote a poem in a form I'd never used before. Part of the form was to start writing only after I felt something beneath the thoughts and language in my head. The feeling couldn't be a memory. It needed to be a real sensation in the moment. Then all the words that followed came in a single sentence, each sentence a simple declaration. For several weeks afterwards I maintained that form in my poems. As I read our poems of this time now, I experience Cathy's words as flow above my one line declarations. I have the image of a small wooden box being filled with water. Perhaps I needed a structure that could contain Cathy's increasingly fluid and free associations. Maybe I needed the sureness of statements declared, rather than asked.

Sixth Chemotherapy

January 29:

I'm up early, excited to see Chris today. We eat breakfast at the Claremont Hotel and go to Tilden Park and ride the trains pulled by steam engines. The 15 gauge is great, but the 7 ½ gauge is really special because it runs only three hours a week, and because there is only seven and a half inches between the wheels, you straddle it. Because of the scale, you go the equivalent of fifty-two miles an hour. If I had hair, it would have been blowing. I feel my life changing scale right now. The track is both wide and narrow, and the pace varied and unknown.

January 30:

It's the day before I go to the doctor. My left eye twitches. No matter how much I try to assure myself all is fine, my body goes into a nervous mode beyond my conscious control.

January 31:

My sixth chemo treatment went well. The chemo oncologist was happy to see me smiling. I guess that is unusual in her world. My feet and hands are close to infection, so I'm supposed to watch them daily, and return if anything changes. I'm babying them as much as possible.

On the aching, she says it's because the white blood cells are fighting so hard. Like every chemo patient, I'm being poisoned, and every two weeks my body fights its way back, hence the reason for the aching. I appreciate that the oncologist is honest. She compares chemo to dying and coming back. She says, "We take you as far as we can, and amazingly, you come back. The human body is amazing." I feel proof of that. It is as though there is some place of wisdom I touch, something old, ancestral, a knowing that there is something big going on here that I, in my rapidly changing bones and cells, can acknowledge and hold.

My oncologist is open about my medical chart. The words, metastasized cancer, glare there. I rarely let myself feel that I am dealing with something big, but I let myself feel that tonight. I understand this is about how I meet the chemo treatment, about how I greet life.

Today was quick, just under five hours by twenty minutes, and relatively painless. The Benadryl dose was cut in half to enable me to rest, instead of having jumpy legs like last time. All the prayers, visualizations and care make a difference. We're counting the days, my blood cells and I. Emerson said, "The earth laughs in flowers." I tap my feet to their beat.

Flight Paths

rain falls outside the window
in the fog and gray light — nothing to see but the tree
huddled, wanting to enter in —
I trim it periodically,
leaning out with shears
so the leaves don't bruise
and crush on glass,
so it doesn't
die like a bird
when it mistakes,
this flight,
for the next —

how does the fog do that
just clear
first nothing
then one tree, then others. climbing the hill, leading my
eyes
like a painting
to a focus
diagonal in intent,
something to climb,
inside, out
and outside, in — mobius strip

— Cathy

94

Each day before Tai Chi we sweep.

The mulberry tree loses its leaves slowly in autumn.
Even during the rainy season its leaves still fall.
Then sweeping is slow.
The wet leaves resist the broom and cling to the ground.
We don't try to clear all the leaves away, then.
In spring, everything is topped in blossom.
We sweep in summer mostly to remember sweeping.

– Jane

Looking Back: Cathy

I woke one late January day, a chemo day, to the healing power of pink light. I felt dipped in the rose shading of the sky. I had been suffering, wanting things to be different than they were, caught in confusion between another's wants and desires and my own. I let it go, cleansed by the pink light of the sky and the ritual of Jane's sweeping.

My surgical scar has been, and continues to be, a gauge. It flames in pain when I seethe in either anger or perceived self-righteousness. Like Harry Potter, I am warned of danger. His danger comes from outside, whereas mine comes from within. I continue to be aware of managing my thoughts, and I understand that judgment is division and does not serve me now. I suffer when I want things to be different than they are. Instead, I can say, "Is that so?" sweep out the old, and make a place for the new.

In the heart of my journey, Jane said I was like a baby, vulnerable, taking everything in whole and at a visceral, cellular level. We were both aware of the need to water grief with tears and allow time to heal. I saw a drawing at this time that looked like a frog when turned one way, and a horse when turned the other. My intention became to open my eyes to see both frog and horse at the same time. That focus was with me as I read Jane's poem. I saw Jane, Jim, and all those who sweep and have swept through time.

Looking Back: Jane

Reading some of Cathy's poems of this time, I'm reminded of the journal I kept when I lived in South Carolina. It documented in twenty-five short poems the eight years my son's father and I struggled to keep our lives together, growing our own food out of necessity, feeling our bond dissolving, not because we'd lost our love, but because we'd lost our way. Most people who read those twenty-five poems never know the pain and struggle that was the ground from which they grew. Rather than being about the sadness of that time, each poem instead represented a brief moment during which I was able to write. Each for me is like a memento pressed in wax. They were the moments when the demands of survival lifted briefly. They were the moments when we'd made some brightness for ourselves to relieve the ache. Still, the words were true, like these words of Cathy's during this time.

Discernment

February 1:

Yesterday, while with the oncologist, I called *Neulasta* 'Neuplasta'. She corrected me, but I think my word works. Feeling tingling in my hands and toes, I Google "neurological" and see what I would rather not know. At times I think I need to know what is going on to visualize, and I also see that it might be best to continue my mantra that the organism is intelligent and knows what to do.

Yesterday a doctor showed some young doctors through the infusion room. The young doctors were self-conscious, and I felt like a zoo specimen, sitting there with my feet up, hooked to an IV, books resting on the table, in an attempt to make my space a home. When I thought of what the word 'infusion' means to me, flowers and flower essences came to mind, with names like Fairy Slippers and Wild Rose. I make each space and situation my own. That is how I cope. I've brought the mountain inside.

Jane said something returned today. I wonder if it is surrender. I sit and infuse, marinate in the touch and movement of cells.

Sea shells

    Doubled,

    clams, oysters, mussels,
    one for each ear.
    I provide
    the sound
    of the sea
    climbing
    in and out
    of spirals
    circling air
    through chambers
    that open
    and meet

    The sea blooms in me.

— Cathy

Dreams trundled through the night.

Like parcels, they arrived at the door of sleep.
Some were filled with flocks of old poets.
They were drinking the rain.
I cupped their dear faces.
Others were as unlikely as this earth.
There were trees without names.
Light, of the kind that is surprising to infants.
When I am old, still I will not know this place.

– Jane

Life-Lines

February 2:

Jane is in Pasadena for work. She calls me at seven from her hotel and listens to my morning flow. She calls it 'Life-Lines'. I am struggling to keep my core, the essential part of my being alive, even as I am probed internally by injections from outside. Last night, I felt invaded by aliens as the chemo searched, like a snake or flashlight, for what rapidly divides. My throat is sore.

As Jane and I talk, I realize I am not looking for meaning in my writing. My mind is unclear, like this day I see outside my window. I record what I see and feel, hoping for an anchor.

I am here. I am me, some me, and sometimes the chemicals cause my legs to shake, and I sit with that. I watch them shake, and this is why, today, I look out the window at the trees and watch them, just watch. I am not looking for meaning, judgment, or even discernment. I just am.

Because the rapidly dividing cells are destroyed with chemotherapy, I continue to celebrate what evolves more slowly in time. I honor the movement in rocks.

Today, there is no meaning, only being, in a life.

The Movement in Rocks

I peel the earth and eat it like an orange,

chew the seeds

welcome the hand that comes like an animal in the night

to write on mind, with porcupine spines,

held at an angle

to catch the light.

— *Cathy*

In the high room of an old hotel, I open windows to the night.

A crescent moon dangles from a palm tree.
From the verandah below, laughter and talk drift up.
As in childhood, I fall asleep to the voices of grownups.
I awaken to birdsong.
It is dawn again, spring again.

How patiently my heart beats.

— Jane

Looking Back: Cathy

When chemo brain, chemo mind, began to wash on through, I scoffed at some of what I had written when I was in treatment. How could I have written that *"I rise like a croissant* and *fluff the moon* and *fold time like dough and feast"*? And yet, it all felt true. I had lived in a magical place. When treatment ended, and the magical place began to disappear and be replaced, the physical reality for me was that I still struggled to enter a grocery store. It was where my stomach balked, and people, noise, and commotion all overwhelmed me. I wondered if I could function in the "real" world as I had before. Where was my place? Could I adjust?

Today I have found balance. Sometimes I pillow and lounge on clouds because I know when they dissipate, I can thrive on the ground. I can part the mist and hold the grail knowing the heart pumps blood both in and out. It circulates and I am free to choose, free to embrace the whole of myself, for as with a tree, there is no front or back. I celebrate that I, like a tree, spread branches 360 degrees around.

Looking Back: Jane

I was on a business trip and staying in a hotel. I'd gone to sleep after working late into the night without completing everything I needed to do. As I fell asleep, and again when I awoke, I was reminded of the experience of falling asleep and waking to the world with the ears of a child. I didn't really want to face the day I had to face. I wanted to linger in contentment, savor a moment of not needing to know, feel nothing but the patient beating of my heart. I wanted to escape into the childhood feeling of safety and constancy.

When I read Cathy words that morning, she was feeling the sensations of a physical rebirth, wanting to know and see everything. Through her willingness to really feel the changes the chemo was making in her, and giving voice to those changes, I experienced briefly that other energy of childhood, an energy that pushes, explores, and wants to know everything. I felt the force it takes to fight for aliveness. I remembered the hunger of childhood, awakening with the desire to eat the world like an orange - seeds and all.

102

Rising from Ashes

February 3:

Yesterday I went to the Cascade Trail with Karena to see the falls on Mt. Tam, and honor her mother and my own. Her mother died last Monday, and mine last year. Next to the pounding waterfall, I read a poem, a gift from Elaine, a poem of the phoenix rising from ashes. My time to grieve for my mother was interrupted when my health became an issue. Today I returned to helping her pass.

Karena said that her mother, in death, looked like a little bird lying there. After my mother's death, I slept in her bed. A glass egg I had given her fell in the night. As I picked up the pieces, I felt her letting me know the egg was broken, and she was flown away, opened to a larger womb. The cardinal she loved sat on her bird-feeder for hours, looking in at me. I took each message to heart.

Unfortunately, the trip to the Cascade trail was a bit much for me, so I came home when I realized my temperature was rising. Steve and I kept monitoring it to make sure I didn't have to go to the hospital. With chemo, the minute it hits 100.5, it's a danger zone, since there aren't enough white blood cells to fight infection. I slept and feel fine this morning, after another lesson in awareness and limitation.

February 4:

Awake at four AM, I observe that my legs are achy and lacking support. There are empty spaces. When I place my foot on the ground, it's not like a pancake spreading, but instead it is a mixture of stones, jagged ones. All is quiet. There is no wind, and the fog is wrapped around like a shawl. The anniversary of my mother's death approaches. Poems come.

103

Healing

I sit among the stones

still and silent

spacious as a field

of Arctic terns

flying pole to pole –

the sea in me is vast

the waves form and reform,

open and close

like the sail

upon the mast.

— Cathy

The Sound of One Hand Clapping

the ashes of mother scattered, tossed, spread in a meadow tended by trees.

the ivory ash, golden in the air, forms images in the evening light

Madonna, Mother and Father, husband and wife, holding hands,

lifted in a cloud-like drift to the woods, the sky, the stream

we sit on a bench

a peal of thunder

the hand clap of one

understood .

— Cathy

Ode to My Mother

When she was here in fragile form,

graceful as the curved spine of Kokopeli,

we rode her gentleness like the back of a whale,

her last words, "so very good,"

as she sipped a glass of chocolate milk.

She holds the portal open so I can see,

bounces me from her hand like a yo-yo

Of time and space I am free.

—Cathy

February 5:

I wake, feeling radiant as though my heart sports a halo from the moistness in all the love I receive. Then there is a shift, and my lack of energy commands the day be one of rest. Mandu agrees, and the day stretches like childhood summer play, sunshine to fireflies. I am fern, awaiting spores.

February 6:

I notice the crescent moons at the base of my nails and see them as smiles. I remember Charlotte Selver, my teacher of Sensory Awareness, saying "Feel the back of your knees as smiles. Let all your cells smile." Lately, I've been feeling like I have no knees. There is no support there, and yet I think it is just a re-arranging of my bones, like pillows on a couch. I form softer smiles.

I am reminded today of the oncology nurse who saw me reading poems and lamented that he was unable to read poetry. He then told me of a complex tradition of Icelandic poems, and spoke of Shakespeare and how any love he might have had was destroyed by having to match passages with speakers in school. He said he wasn't taught in school that poems were about real people and feelings. He continued to lament that he didn't know poetry, and that it had been taken from him, and he was too old to return. He didn't realize he was a bard, the oral tradition revived, as he told stories to me.

I continue to feel this as an opportunity to return to childhood, when we were both young and old at the same time because we were so aware of growth. Each day something was gained and something left behind. We measured progress daily, able to climb another step, fit into a bigger swing, and leave the smaller swing behind.

I go to the dentist, where I am warmly greeted and hugged. I say this experience is a gift, and my dentist understands. She and her husband wanted children, but it was not to be, and they learned through that to appreciate life in a whole new way. They found a gift in their pain, and because of my experience with this, I am able to connect with her and what she has gained.

February 7:

I read Joan Didion's, The Year of Magical Thinking. She writes of grief and how it comes in waves, and of her mother, who, in her 90's, did not want to leave her children, who were in their 60's, because she felt they still needed her. I continue to consider non-attachment as I work to see death as just a step. I know that those I love, all of you, are doing fine, and my passing through the veil may leave you feeling waves, waves of pain, and also, with reflection, understanding and joy. And of course, at this point, there is no knowing who goes first.

It is recorded by St. Luke that Christ and the Apostles sat at a circular table during the Last Supper. From that may have come the legend and myth of King Arthur and the Round Table. I am attracted to that idea of equality right now, the notion of integrating each segment of treatment in a circle, honoring the meeting of head and tail, the beginning and end undefined.

My dining room table is circular. I used it when I cooked today, making a real meal, chopping onion, ginger, and garlic. When I opened the cupboard to peer within, I realized I have not been able to face herbs and spices this whole time, but today, I did. Our meals have been rather plain so I was delighted to invite new foods to play. Taxol is not about nausea, and it has taken me awhile to believe that, but it seems the change has begun. Steve has never complained; he has remained a master of presence, a soothing Zen teacher for me.

February 8:

Steve and I walked around the block this morning enjoying Venus, and the sky was noticeably brighter a little earlier today. Years ago, I attended a memorial service at a beautiful home on Mount Tam. At the door was an open bowl filled with daffodil bulbs for each of us to take as we left. I took five and buried them in a pot on the deck. Those daffodils are up once again, yellow flags announcing the return of spring.

108

February 9:

One thing I have appreciated was that, though it had thinned, I still had a soft, fluffy triangle of pubic hair. Yesterday, I noticed it was really thin, and today, it is gone, dropped down the drain. I sit with that. I am sad. Pubic hair is a symbol of womanhood, and it's odd to have it gone. I wonder if it will return, and for now, it is not here, and so it is. It is another confirmation of change. Sometimes I think I'm imagining this whole thing, and then, I see I am hairless. I can see myself as either alien, or swept clean. I see the female child, exposed.

February 10:

Elaine sends an email saying I should be thrilled. I have a Brazilian Bikini Wax. So now, I am "hip" and "in." Who would have thought? I enjoy a class with Daniel Polikoff in my continuing study of Rilke. I learn that in the words, "Blessed are the meek," *meek* means pure of soul.

When chemo sends my pubic hair flowing down the drain,
I learn I have a Brazilian bikini wax
without the expense or pain... somewhat.

I revel in the physical realm, Bread, the spiritual, Wine,
the life force, Milk, the soul, Honey, evolving like rich, golden
swirls made from pollen, the movement of bees.

The princess in fairy tales stands for the soul,
yearning, longing, a place to fill, a cauldron,
and mine is filled with laughing frogs, toads and newts

cavorting in a hot tub, jubilant as chorus girls.
Death may draw us in, like life,
tapped syrup poured from trees.

— Cathy

Of all the places in the world, here is most mysterious.

Sometimes I am alone here.
Other times, you, your feet up the steps, the door
opening.

Then our words become tomorrow before the sounds
have left our lips.
When there are stars, here is invisible.
In the light, it is everything.

– Jane

Looking Back: Cathy

My pubic hair has returned. In those days, I was on a swing, tossed from tears to exuberance like a child. This was my "good" week of the two. I understood more and more that life is a continuum and I was living with the tides, flowing in and out. When I read Aldous Huxley's words on his experience with mescaline, I recognized a piece of the chemo experience, a place of bliss where nothing matters or holds together, where seeing is "what Adam had seen on the morning of his creation – the miracle, moment by moment, of naked existence." "Neither agreeable nor disagreeable," Huxley said. "It just is."

I was surprised that the loss of the pubic hair was so unsettling. Perhaps it was because I wasn't prepared. Or, perhaps it brought back those days of my first period and the welcoming into womanhood, which now seemed very fragile in comparison as I appeared to dwell in an androgynous state, unable to discern male or female, or good or bad, in this complex, yet simple place.

Looking Back: Jane

Cathy was undergoing physical transformation and living every day in her body. To me, she seemed to sit with the unknown, easily and with openness. She found analogies that stood in for the mute, 'un-languaged' experience of being. For me, living mostly in the world of work, my world was defined by what could be seen and named. Somehow, by living in this concrete world, the idea of "here" was gone before I knew it. Most of my time was tied to 'doing'. That the infinite lives always and forever, all at once, was a concept that I could often feel during the morning writing with Cathy, but it would quickly dissolve as my day began. For me, Cathy's choices in dealing with her illness embodied, in addition to the pain and worry, a kind of embracing of jubilance, as well as living "the miracle, moment by moment, in naked existence." It was a well I came to every morning. Gradually, I think the thirst it quenched in me lasted a little bit longer each day, and carried me a little bit farther into the world.

Seventh Chemotherapy

February 12:

The word February derives from *februare,* meaning to purify, to cleanse. It looks like that from here. The plum trees are cheerleaders of spring with their pompom blossoms. I feel well. I am learning to rest. Steve and I walked down for coffee and saw the sun pop us as the earth turned.

I would like to talk about death. It seems some who read my blog wonder why I speak so often about death. I'm actually quite joyful as I am coming to an acceptance, or perhaps, an understanding of the cycle of life and death in which we all live. It's like the water cycle, constantly in motion. Right now, it's so obvious to me because I feel cells dying, observing, participating, hanging out, growing, renewing. I'm all the seasons at one time. I'm budding, growing, losing leaves, and am dormant all at once. I am a hot-house flower, whipping through bloom after bloom. I'm the sea, resplendent with tides. Someone asked me yesterday if my oncologist had prescribed anti-depressants. I said no; she feels a person would be nuts not to feel depressed at times like this. I feel it; I honor it, and away it goes, swooshing out with a glide.

My mother feels close as I honor the anniversary of her death. Would I embrace each sunrise in the same way if I were immortal? As I become more comfortable with death, I'm more aware of life. I continue to birth.

Jeff, Jan, and I drove to Point Reyes to consider Heart's Desire Beach as a location for their wedding. We ate in the garden of the Station House Café. It is my first trip there since this happened, and in the past, it was my ritual. I came to Pierce Point each week after my mother died, feeling her there. I balance now on a seesaw, feeling death, and in that, appreciating life. The full moon rises as clouds flow like veils.

February 13:

Jane tells me about a man who is getting his Ph.D. in "Deliciousness" at UCSF. He's studying neuroscience from the point of view of what makes something delicious. Yum!

Jeff and I checked out more places for a wedding today. I am encouraging elopement. I prepare for chemo tomorrow, Valentine's Day. I will certainly get a deep shot of Cupid's arrow.

February 14:

Today is my seventh chemo day. I don't seem too nervous. My eye isn't twitching, so I'm taking that as a good sign. I find myself singing, "Happiness is only two more chemo treatments." I float into infusion world and all goes reasonably well. As usual, it's hard to get the needle in, and I feel the chemo swirl. I am thrilled to be nearing the end. I realize this is how people get through wars. We respond to an end.

Everyone is cheerful today because it is Valentine's Day. It seems the side effects with my feet and glowing head are most unusual. I may be the only one. As I leave, I'm very cheerful because now I ONLY HAVE ONE MORE CHEMO TREATMENT. This is so exciting, I can hardly stand it, and I do. We go out to dinner to celebrate.

February 15:

There is an article in the *New York Times* today on the cost of the drug Avastin, which is used to treat cancer. The current cost is $100,000 a year. Some insurance companies are balking at the cost. Sometimes it only increases life by a few months. Other times, it is effective, but much is unproven. Because the producers of Avastin are charging such a high price, the fear is that other companies will do the same for other drugs.

I'll have my shot of Neulasta today. It costs $5000.00, and I will have had eight of them by the time I'm finished. My insurance is covering the cost, but what if it weren't? What if we had to come up with that kind of money? Could we? Where does it stop? Now that I am so intimately connected with the cost of cancer treatment, I'm paying more attention. It's another moral issue with which to wrestle: "How do we divide this pie we share?"

Morning Light

the wind has passed
the day is quiet
who would know the chairs
were blown over in the night
that I awakened in disquieting fright
concerned for the pines overhead -
now
there is nothing to say
if I listen to the day
all was said
before
the light

— *Cathy*

Sometimes the human heart is a woman in a red dress.

It calls down a long hallway, "You loved me once, once, once."
Sometimes it drinks its own sorrows into a ragged gulping sleep.
Like a harlot, it's been known to entertain its doubts deep into the night.
And yet, even alone and at a distance, it can feel into the dark.
And when it is as ripe as a persimmon, sweet with autumn love,

Even blindfolded, it can know the heart of other hearts.

— Jane

115

Looking Back: Cathy

I was awakening to the financial costs of my treatment, which even though covered, still meant I was using a huge piece of the shared pie. On the other hand, this treatment regimen is experimental, is research, so what is discovered through my treatment will benefit others. I continued to be aware I was part of a tribe, an expensive link at this point, and yet one that seemed to matter. I was a welcome partner on the lifeboat planet, Earth.

I missed my mother and I was part of planning a wedding. It was a time to continue balancing involvement and rest, life and death.

Looking Back: Jane

I'm usually drawn more to the bones and earth, drawn to the essence, to the color that lasts in the dried bloom, the truth that lives in the shape of our bodies and our faces as experiences move through us. Still, I do know and feel the passion of the pungent wind, the lightning, the shock of snow that turns us blind, the rush of chemicals, blood, and adrenaline as we connect with others. I know within myself that these are the forces that move life through me. But my hope is that passion is more than the flash of "the woman in the red dress." My hope is that passion's nature has as much to do with what happens after that flash, and with the transformation occurs. Where am I left when the passion has run through me? Being there daily with Cathy's illness and the real possibility of dying has led me to hope that when it is my time to leave, my heart will be like the flesh of the fruit ripened by all that passed through it, that I will have become who I am in essence, and that my love will, like the stone and flesh of the fruit, be given back.

Remember to Look

February 16:

Chemo has struck again. Today, it has gone for my tongue, which is swollen and thick.

The shot I receive the day after chemo should be given over five to ten days, but because it is too much for people to drive there every day, it is given in one blast. I think of the cave days where the herbalist-shaman-healer lived nearby, to give a daily dose. And yet, what if a mammoth ate the healer or the local herb supply dried up? There is always risk. How do I balance what I can reasonably do around my health with feelings of peace, ease, and well-being? Perfection is static. I allow movement and change, and try to catch the still point, honor the pause, the place between.

Jane calls this morning from a hotel. She is on a business trip and missing home. I miss knowing she is close.

Winter Life

The rose in February waits, protected by thorns
while fairies knit caps and caterpillar shoes,
to warm the light,
until, like a wand, the sun with its rays
opens petals and butterflies,
and there, what rested, is born from night.

— Cathy

Day breaks the roof of this old building.

The ceiling cracks reveal its many lives.

Water and heat and elevators plunge through its arteries.
Here footsteps hurry down a fire escape, though nothing is
burning.
There the bed is bottomless.
The linens are whiter than the china or the hands of laundry
ladies.

Those who live here, do not sleep here.
Those who sleep here cannot hear the stories in the walls.

– Jane

118

On a Rough Chemo Day

I am caught on points of pain
as chemo like Drano
runs through my drain.
All hair is gone.
Tongue, hands, feet,
organs and bones are sore.
I am given a chance to come back,
to grow new hair and cells that float like boats
in this ocean that seems to be me,
and I, it.

Every day I am grateful
for the gift of that.
I look up at the sky
its guidance a hook
and climb the stones inside
the jewels placed there
when I pause and slow
and remember to remember,
to look.

— Cathy

Remembrance

I pick young Rosemary today

to layer with chicken, carrots,

garlic, potatoes -

The tendrils are soft curls.

They lie there,

> *remember,*

> *the vine.*

— Cathy

It was so brief.

> *Our sleeves just barely touched as I passed.*
> *I didn't notice.*
> *Then from behind, "Excuse me."*
> *Like a voice through anesthesia.*
>
> *Then louder,*
> *"The lesson for today is excuse me."*
> *Like a lover spurned.*
> *I turned.*
> *Our eyes met.*
> *There was the human face of history's hungry fee.*
> *There was where the damage lay.*
>
> *My courage nearly failed, and then,*
> *"I'm sorry."*

– Jane

Looking Back: Cathy

My job was simple. Notice; receive; appreciate. I was letting go and seeding new growth. Chemo allowed me to be aware of birthing and dying, battling and renewing, destroying and growing, all at the same time. Pregnant with change, I lived in pause and in an emptiness that expands.

There were days my tide was low, rocks were exposed, and my organism shrank from the light of the sun, and yet, no matter what, I could go out into my yard and pick rosemary, the symbol of remembrance, and inhale the fragrance and layer its nutrients in my food. In those winter days, I was wrapped in wool, looking through gauze, living enclosed. Summer and Independence Day were yet to come.

Looking Back: Jane

During this time, I was in a class about diversity and racism. It was difficult for me. I didn't talk about it much. I remember feeling resistance and a little sick on the days I had the class. It was — it is — hard to look at the ways our culture has evolved and to realize that I, too, have contributed to the pain. But I understand now as I look back, reading the words of those days in February, that part of what Cathy's and my mornings together have given me is a daily practice of experiencing what another being brings to this moment, and to feel that experience as a real sensation in my body, not just in my thoughts. I know a bit more now about what it feels like standing in another's shoes.

Letting Go

February 18:

I'm awakened by moonlight. The pain probes through the Ibuprofen, so I rise with the moon and make waffles. Today is the anniversary of my mother's death. Jan Chiaramonte gives me the gift of a handmade quilt. I am touched and amazed that she would make a quilt for me, so beautiful and perfect, and that it would come *this* day. She met me only once, at her son's wedding, and yet she knows what I need. Tonight I sit by the fire under my new quilt. Mother Love comes through many people and in many forms.

February 19:

It's a lazy Sunday morning. Chris is here and we each seem to be in our own little cocoon of silence. My knees are tingly. I'm certain I'm in the process of being remade as a kangaroo or gazelle. I'm thinking I would like some hair. I tap my head, feel the cranial bones, and honor the continents that shift in and out, up and down, the movement that comes with breath.

February 20:

I wiggle inside. It's light at seven a.m. as we write. The sun returns. It is not like living on the equator here. We live with seasonal changes of light. Yesterday I saw each Redwood branch hold a clear water ball, an ornament, a capsule of rain. I think we do that with memories when we roll them on our tongue, rather than letting them fall.

Rice Paddies

"In Balinese language and understanding, 'rice paddies' equals 'jewel' equals 'mind.'"

Stewart Brand writing on a talk by Stephen Lansing

In Bali, the music is dense

like their view of time,

which overlaps,

ten kinds of weeks concurrently,

solar, lunar, seven-day, six-day on down

to a one-day week.

We view time as past, present, future,

linear; each day is strapped to a rod we climb,

looking back or up, at what we've done,

and what is yet to do.

When I try and stretch my mind

to view this day ten ways,

I hear the squeak of the rising of the sun,

the setting down of the moon,

the roar and purr of clouds,

the lifting of dew.

I see the hills and trees

from top to bottom

reflected underneath,

124

by worms carving,

gophers mounding,

and moles tunneling

deeply below.

And I'm spun like a top,

on the whirr of blood and leaves,

exchanging gases,

like letters,

as pollen is carried

by bees.

— Cathy

I woke in the night.

Light pooled in the corner of the room.
A twitch electrified my spine.
I found I had grown a pelt of quills.
Uprooting one, I dipped it into ink.
It drew a fine true line
Sliced the moon in half.
In the morning, frost on all the blossoms.

— Jane

February 21:

I am feeling well in the moment. This last week has been a rough one, and I'm glad to feel the chemo moving through. I'm sad though, to now also lose my eyebrows and eyelashes. It's one more letting go, and perhaps it is more efficient to have more room on my face. During the day, I feel happy, as though wallabies bounce in me, making juice from fruit. I also feel the tree outside call to me asking me to feel what rubs inside the movement of the leaf. In doing that, I lean to feel the trunk holding *me* up and see what the leaf may or may not see, and realize when we don't feel and honor that stalk of support, we may feel lonely and grieve. In the evening, I am tired and remember the effects are cumulative. I settle in to rest.

February 22:

I woke this morning, grateful for life, all life. Waves of gratitude flow through me. I am in a place of non-judgment, just being. I have no words, and I know it won't last, but if this is one of the gifts of chemo, it's so worth it. As Rumi says, "There are many ways to kneel and kiss the ground." I'm learning to rest when I need to rest, and I have the luxury of that right now. I'm also learning not to fight the fatigue or judge it, and though sometimes I do, I continue to simmer in acceptance and change. The words that come right now are gratitude, appreciation, immersion, awe, and love. My heart is more than a heart. My trunk is aglow. The early morning sun touches the hill and then me. I am lit, pulled out of the carriage house and attached to the horse. I give thanks.

Evolving Dew as It Forms
> *The trees wake,*
> *See the ponds within*
> *pearls formed not from wounds*
> *but begun uniform as a drop of dew*
> *which is how the ancients thought pearls*
> *were formed.*

— Cathy

126

Today's poem.

I have in front of me an absolutely blank page.

-   Jane

Looking Back: Cathy

I was grateful Jane gave herself permission to write a non-poem. She had been steady in this process. I thought she deserved a break. I was glad she was letting go.

I, aware of overlap, ran my fingers over the round circle of the crescent moon, aware there was more than I saw, and I listened as though to a finger on the rim of a crystal glass.

I sat, eyes closed, recognizing that though we say the sun rises and sets, it is the earth that turns and revolves. Our axis tilts. How do we miss so much of the dance? Is there more than we are able to ingest, the world so prolific, entertaining and abundant, that sometimes in our awe, we close our eyes in retreat?

Roots intertwine in more ways than we realize as Mother Earth provides a home. I was learning to trust in letting go.

Looking Back: Jane

On the day the page went blank and no words urged themselves into my fingers, I heard in a different way. Something shifted for me as Cathy and I talked. The months of writing together, every morning, no matter what, about whatever, had brought me to this place where I found myself listening — not for the wound, not for the story — but for the place where I dropped from nothing into nothing, like dew entering rain, or rain entering the ocean. I realized Cathy and I could sit together in silence. I felt we had arrived at a new level of confidence in one another, and at a whole new place in our friendship. Allowing myself a morning of just *being* without doing was new for me.

Preparing for Radiation

February 23:

I wake feeling well and give myself a cheer, then write about the crescent moon beaming in the sky, and know just *that* can be enough excitement for a day. I see the sun touch a section of needles on the redwood tree, inviting a color of green I've never seen before. Now I understand why some say the moon is made of green cheese. "Say cheese," said the crescent moon to the tree, and the tree reflected back green and the smile of *cheese* to the moon.

I had an appointment at 1:00 today with the radiation oncologist, Dr. Francine Halberg. I went to the Cancer Institute calm, confident, and alone, thinking, "I am used to this stuff by now. I don't need anyone to go with me." Wrong!

I was asked to update my forms for chemo and was happy to see that when I began chemo, I checked a six on a scale of one to ten for anxiety. Today, feeling perfect ease, I checked a one. My blood pressure was normal. Francine popped into the room, and my eyes widened as I looked at her bright red hair and huge blue eyes. Again, I was surprised as my idea of what a doctor is 'supposed to' look like changed. She looked like a movie star. We talked and loving my attitude, she said I would do super at radiation.

She also said she had just attended a conference, and new findings showed that I needed another operation to remove more lymph nodes. "No way," I said, "I'm not healed from the last one." She went through the statistics and said I had a few days to make a decision, and if I refused the operation, I would be targeted extra hard with radiation.

I was feeling a bit unsettled at this point, so I decided to mention that when I took my shower, I noticed my breast was slightly red and swollen. She checked and now it was red and hard as a rock. She called for a sonogram and I walked to another building for a procedure that turned out to be the most painful experience of my life. The numbing didn't work and the practitioner went in with a needle over and over again. I was shaking and crying. I left at six, and still had to stop to fill a prescription for antibiotics.

Ever had a day where you felt like you were being tested? I don't understand the percentages and statistics, but today I heard there is an eight percent chance this will recur no matter what I do. That, plus my

129

three percent chance of dying from other causes, means an eleven percent chance that I will die and now, I ask myself, "By what date?" since I am very clear there is a *one hundred percent certainty* I am going to die.

I noticed today the new meditation garden is finished. I appreciate that people are doing all they can to save me, and at some point, I think we all need to face we are going to die. That can't be changed.

Oddly, when the pus was being painfully removed from the abscess, I was told how much better I would feel. I hadn't even noticed that I wasn't feeling okay. I am so used to discomfort that it hadn't registered that something was wrong. Today I was focused on the pain in my feet. I am reminded of my oncologist's words, "There are no good days in chemo." I see there are varying degrees of discomfort, but there is always something there.

The problem probably occurred because the blood vessel from the biopsy is weakened, so any touch can cause a problem. The good news is that now I'm on antibiotics, so I should do fine in going to see Rachel Naomi Remen Saturday night. We haven't been to a movie, and I haven't been in a group since chemo began, but I want to see her with Steve, Jeff, and Jan.

I arrived home to an email from the friend who gave me the quilt. "You know," she wrote, "I believe the quilt nearly made itself for you. I asked Thom to check with Steve about your favorite colors and the answer was 'earth tones'. I went to a large fabric outlet in Orange County where I shop frequently, and came to these flannels within five minutes of being in the store. I decided when I saw the fabric that I would quilt leaves, flowers, and grasses in the squares. All of that is to say that your quilt was meant to be."

February 24:

I wake feeling I've been run over by a truck. I also feel support. Jeff and Chris will come by today. Either or both would have gone with me yesterday. I had only to ask. Steve would have stayed in town. Jane, too, says she would have taken a vacation day to come and support me. Others have offered over and over again to help. I'm still working on believing I'm not a bother, and that people consider it a gift to be allowed to help me. People want to be part of this process. How can they receive the pleasure of giving if I am not able to receive? Slowly, painfully, I learn.

A Haiku of Tears

Everything seems sad -

The daffodils need watering.

The sun is out –

— Cathy

The place where two elevated highways join had made a roof.

Beneath, an island in the middle of two streets.

There, briefly, was a bed made up like home.
Blankets cornered. Pillow fluffed. A teddy bear.
As if the walls had blown away.
Leaving only roof and floor
And that proud bed.

– Jane

Looking Back: Cathy

This was a tough time, even though I comforted myself with knowing that tears form rainbows, and rain brings tulips and daffodils, and a bed can be a home no matter where that bed is made. I kept hearing the words of Masahide: "My house burned down. I can now see better, the rising moon."

A year later, my breast was still sore and swollen, and yet I preferred the extra dose of radiation to another operation, which would have given me another twelve percent, but twelve percent of what, I have no idea. I never understood the statistics, but I was slowly learning how much people love to give, and how much more acceptance and reception of that there was for me to learn to receive.

Looking Back: Jane

How sensitive we can be, as humans, how seemingly unfit for life; how challenging it is to watch ourselves passing through time and space, knowing our own births and deaths. How mere are the words we have to tell this tale; how driven we are to try to capture the dialog, see the pattern, name the thing, share with others. How brave and foolish we are. How much we depend on hope.

Maybe it is easier not to notice that we live with tears in our eyes. We survive in the face of pain and loss and loneliness and shunning. But after five months of mornings, I'd found I had expanded my capacity for standing with the wonder of being here for *all* of it, of finding my way new every day, of witnessing my own daily transformation and of sharing that with Cathy.

A Place to Rest

February 25:

Fog rolls over the hills and curves. The infection is alive in my breast, and I feel well. I shed some tears and find in my morning poem that twelve bumblebees come and ask if they can ride on my shoulders. I walk to the ocean with them as guests, and when we arrive, they gasp and ask what it means. I say, "It's where we all come clean."

February 26:

Yesterday, Jane and I met in person for the first time since we began writing together. We wanted to look back at what I had written about the surgery and the beginning of chemo. I had been avoiding looking back, but was surprised to find it was not shocking. I was barely touching the surface with my words. I was like a water strider cohering to the surface of the pond, while whirlpools raged below. I see that we self-protect, and I know we can't heal what we can't feel, so I again look to the writing to help me more earnestly probe what is now ready to be revealed.

I'm concerned about my red and white blood cells now that the abscess is still a problem, and I am fighting off a cold and the flu.

I loved hearing Rachel Naomi Remen speak, and Jan bought me her book, *Kitchen Table Wisdom*, and when Rachel autographed it, she said how blessed I was to have a future daughter-in-law who loves me so much. Before Rachel spoke, a man who had just been through chemo sang some songs he had written. The first one was on how people kept saying to him, "Only two more weeks of chemo." Though his song was an attempt to cheer, I see the end will be worse than I thought.

Rachel learned she had Crohn's Disease when she was fifteen. She was told she would be dead before the age of forty. She is now 68. She has had operations and utilized medical science and she spoke of the will to live as key, and of the mystery and importance of intuition. She was speaking primarily to a group of medical professionals and she said that life is "outside the box," and most medical professionals think so strongly inside the box, they cannot even imagine outside. She helped me decide not to do the second operation. My will to live is strong. It is enough.

On Thursday, while waiting for my radiation oncology appointment, I heard what I thought was a symphony of Tibetan bells, gongs, drums. I was reveling in the harmony, when I realized it was jackhammers at the entry to the building. The sounds expanded out into the atrium and I perceived what I needed to in the moment; I found comfort in making the sound my own. Sometimes I hear the freeway as the ocean, or a rushing stream. It is up to me to give myself what I need. Again, it is a reminder to learn to receive.

February 27:

It rained through the night, and I reveled in dreams of being in Mexico and swimming in warm ocean waters. Mandu was there, and we swam like sea otters. My mother was there, lively as could be, and said she had found a ride.

My surgeon Allison was appalled when she saw my breast. She blames the problem on the practitioner who did the 'procedure'. All that was needed was a needle check to see if there was an infection. Now, the skin is infected. Anyway, she prescribed two antibiotics, since the first one did nothing, and she wants to see me in a week. She says no chemo tomorrow. I'm delayed at least a week. I'm disappointed and exhausted, even though I know it's the best thing. So there is no celebration of the last day of chemo tomorrow, and there is no celebration of a week off, since antibiotics mean no alcohol. What a journey!

Jane is in New York this week at a search engine conference. Dedicated as always, she writes today's poem on her Blackberry amidst a thousand search engine developers, marketers, and vendors. I would like wider travels, and yet, I know that "wherever I go, there I am," so this is fine too. I journey within.

Why Not Me?

We might ask, "Why me?"

but if we say "Why me?" to everything

where is our facet of the diamond

our chance to climb steep slopes

and slide back down?

Why not me?

Give me every experience

every chance to place my axe

to anchor my boots.

I rise to see

sunrise after sunrise

and descend to bring

sunset to rest

like a fire

banked for the night

in me.

— Cathy

Blackberry Poem from the Search Engine Conference

　A thousand people
　Who spend millions on one word.
　Never tell a poet
　Words are cheap.

– Jane

Looking Back: Cathy

I was intrigued with the Search Engine Conference, and the money spent to locate the one word that would make an advertisement click and move it to the top of the search engine list. A poet also searches for a particular word, though the reward is spiritual, and rarely financial. One word can tap a reader awake. A poet wants to find that word and use it just the right way. For me, poetry is an attempt to write of the forest before the trees. In this journey, I was doing the same thing, imagining a world I could build where each event would rise solid and strong as a tree.

Looking Back: Jane

I work with computers for a living, but have, at best, a cautious optimism, and frequent ambivalence about computer technology. As Cathy and I were able to continue our connection in spite of distance, me with just a Blackberry, she limited by the regimen of treatments, my ambivalence leaned a little more towards the positive. Computers and the web have allowed many people, not just those with access to radio or TV stations and publishing houses, to report on their lives. Might this ability also allow us to see ourselves instantly within the context of "all of us"? Might it be possible that accessible and widespread communication could frame the suffering each one of us experiences as only a small part of the suffering of the world? Could this provide us - me - the perspective of that context? Could this shared consciousness allow us to experience what Naomi Shihab Nye speaks to in her poem "Kindness":

> You must wake up with sorrow.
> You must speak to it till your voice
> catches the thread of all sorrows
> and you see the size of the cloth.
> Then it is only kindness that makes sense anymore.

Care

February 28:

This morning, I wake at 4:00 a.m., and rise at 5:00 a.m. I seem to be on New York time with Jane.

Cat Mandu hops up on my white nightgown with muddy feet. He is scared and needs to snuggle. I notice he is drinking less water, so he needs to go out less.

Jane spoke yesterday about the "emotional price of a given word", and how much advertisers pay to search and research *the* word that will draw us in. Imagine if *we* paid that kind of attention to every word we thought or said, choosing our words as carefully as our finest poets. Imagine a world where words chosen by us, swirl up from within, not influenced by marketers who use words for profit and gain.

We had hail, rain, sun, thunder and lightning, more hail, more rain, and a power outage this morning. It reflects my life. Many people called this morning, many of them from the medical community. They care and are so apologetic about the mishap with the 'procedure'. None of this is their fault, and yet they act as though it is. Again, I am touched.

My many doctors are agreed on no chemo today. I have a staph infection and am on two antibiotics, so hopefully all will clear, and next Tuesday, I will have my final chemo and a celebration. I am both disappointed and elated to not have chemo for a week.

All the visualizing everyone has done for my red and white blood cells worked. My blood tested normal yesterday. Now I'm asking friends to visualize the staph infection gone, and my breast as normal and healthy as can be.

Tender

Each word hung on a line with other words —

speak only kindness —

what else do we need —

The embers of the fire

fall apart.

Air spires the heart

climbs on sparks to see the arc

of landing

each word

as prayer —

— Cathy

Avenue of the Americas

Holding open the door to my heart for each passing face.
When did we divide the human race?

I wake up in a new country.

The streets are paved in salt.

Breakfast is a single egg.

An unfamiliar tune

Bells, a woodwind
Make me homesick.

– Jane

Looking Back: Cathy

In New York, at the Search Engine Conference, Jane studied the importance of a word, one word. In that place of struggle for dominance and hierarchy, she noticed each face. I wanted to feel and label sorrow, fear, anger, and hope, and fly those feelings like kites, mobiles, tender in the air, open to the light.

I wasn't interested in the story of how the feelings were built, just how they might float for awhile, entertain, pass, and quietly disappear. I wanted to honor and follow the change.

Six months later, Jane returned to the Search Engine Conference, this time in San Jose. At the west coast conference, there was a session about people who had blogged about their medical conditions and how much that blogging had helped them. Though I often felt isolated and worried I was falling behind, I was pleased to know I was actually in the flow, modern, and up-to-date.

Steve was on his way to Finland. Through 'Virtual Finland', I learned that Finns place great value on words and choose them carefully. They believe in the Chinese proverb, "Your speech should be better than silence; if not, be silent."

Originally, communication was non-verbal. Then a grunt accompanied the pointing hand. Now, messages are exchanged, ten fingers flying, communicating almost immediately what is thought and felt. One tap of a button and we send and receive. People clump through blogs in the same way that cells unite into organs, heart, liver, lungs. We are learning new ways to band and bond, and in that, we need to remember that each word is precious, and that hurled words can hurt bones more painfully than sticks and stones.

Looking Back: Jane

How do we comfort one another from inside our own pain?

Sometimes my stories wrap around me. Sometimes they pass through me like all those faces on the street. Sometimes stories are a small fire I sit beside. They melt my heart. Then they are just a line of words, and when I have laid the last of the lines on the fire, I am warm for a moment. Sometimes, after the story is done, one word, or one face, remains glowing and true. How many of the stories and faces who pass can I really feel? Even if it is unfamiliar, can I let it transform me?

Healing Hands

March 1:

At seven a.m. my time, Jane heads to MOMA in NYC, and asks what I want to see. I go online to see what's there, and as I roam, she finds "The House of Spiritual Retreat," by Emilio Ambasz. He imagined a site and designed the house on the imaginary site. Then he actually found the site he'd imagined, and built his house. It was built in 2004 "on a hilly, arid landscape outside of Seville."

Jane then finds Van Gogh's "Olive Trees". While she is looking at the painting in the museum, she talks to me on the phone, and I look at the painting online. Yoshio Taniguchi, the architect of the renovated MOMA in NYC, said, "If you raise really a lot of money, I will make the architecture disappear." Isn't that our hope for a poem?

Jane leaves soon for Spain. We begin to prepare for an end to our morning calls while she is gone. For now, even when she is in NY, we talk. Though most of her poems written in NY are sent by Blackberry, and are therefore, short, she sends this poem to me. I know we are connected in a way that she will let me know what she sees. We come together and part, like healing hands.

Let me tell you what I saw.

Not exactly saw but felt.

A hill along a river was encircled by olive trees.

There two white walls, two stories tall, came together in a vee.

At the top where they joined there was one window.

It opened out onto a Spanish balcony.

Like a doll's house, the insides were exposed.

Stairways ascended to the single window.

One along the flank of each tall wall.

The house was buried in the ground beneath those ladders.

Kiva-like, it was full of daylight from a window in its earth-roof.

A common space faced the pure privacy of rooms in slumber,

A palapa looking out into a well of light

Bounced within a plastered gully

Unroofed and gulping in the thick blue sky.

It was a lone house in the Andalucian countryside.

A flame in the darkness, a cave in the heat.

Designed for a landscape imagined before it was found

Like a poem at a loss for words.

— Jane

March 2:

My mother comes to me in a dream. I carry a child, and slip down a slide with the child in my arms. I feel my mother carrying me, her sweet smile. We go back and forth exchanging roles, mother and child. One tear comes, just one. It is enough. I feel full and empty at the same time.

March 3:

I actually feel well. It's amazing. I have breath. My shoulders are back and down. They are no longer earmuffs. My feet are still numb and tingling, and not able to easily welcome shoes, but I am refreshed enough to smile and wiggle my toes and begin to prance. There are rainbows everywhere as the sun and rain play peek-a-boo and bow, curtsy, and dance.

March 4:

I wake at 4:00 a.m., read, and then fall back to sleep, and dream of teaching people they can have fun with cancer, chemo and radiation. Hmmm! What does this dream mean?

March 6:

Morning:

Jane and I talk and I tell her how frightened I am. I feel bloody, sad, and bruised. I am surprised to feel alone. All through this, I have felt support. Perhaps I fear the unknown, the radiation machine. I envision it as huge, and me as a drop under a microscope. Perhaps I am well enough to feel fear. There is no need to pretend, to keep a straight spine. I don't have to say, "I'm fine." I look out on a beautiful day, and tears gather like clouds. Mortality is up for me today, allowing me to appreciate this day even more.

Evening:

Even though I still have infection, and will continue with two antibiotics, I am approved for chemo tomorrow. I am grateful to finish chemo, and all agree I need a break, so I won't see the radiation oncologist for two weeks, or the surgeon for three. That will set me up for radiation to begin, but for now, I just have to finish chemo and rest.

After the rain, the earthworms.

Drowned and thirsty they undertook their blind pilgrimage
Across the concrete to an unknown destiny.
I was the hand of a lesser god
And laid them in the gentle grass.
Though small, I could do this.

— Jane

Looking Back: Cathy

I needed very little, and yet one day I bought a hand-sewn, soft leather hat from the woman who made it. I needed a hand upon my head, the woman's hand, Jane's.

I was beginning to see how hard this was on Jane. I felt I was the earthworm and Jane had lifted me and placed me gently in the grass. Though small, she had done this. Her influence was huge.

Looking Back: Jane

One day in my poem, an omnipotent hand appeared and rescued a worm. I don't know about the earthworm's nervous system, but I imagine that the hand of rescue, even as it saves the worm from its watery grave, may feel like fear.

The other day, a friend took Jim and me to a Native American flute concert. R.C. Nakai, who has advanced the resurgence of Native American flute music in the U.S., spoke and played. He spoke of fear and of its strong hold on the world. He advocated flute playing as an antidote to fear. His words reminded me of something Cathy has often said about fear, that it is excitement without the breath. The notion that flute playing - and poetry - could heal our world by adding breath to fear no longer seems so abstract to me.

Last Chemotherapy

March 7:

This is the day of my last chemo treatment, number eight. How could one describe it? Excitement Ho!

The Morning of My Last Chemo Treatment

I dress carefully and well, wrap around my wrist
a pink breast cancer watch
and a healing bracelet with beads
of Jade, African Jade, Amethyst,
Yellow Jade, Turquoise,
Averturine Red, and Jasper.
I'm cozy in a white turtleneck sweater,
scented with Romance,
and accented with a blue and gold waterfall
flowing from and around my neck.
A rose-quartz angel fills my pocket.
I am fresh, clean, arranged for infusion.
My skin is soft, eyes are open.
The slow-growing cells thank me this morning
for this chance to grow and explore.
They feel honored.
The fast will come back, or not.
The tortoise is out of the shell
and has learned
to hop.

— *Cathy*

How do I describe the joy of my last chemo day? My nurses gave me a graduation ceremony and a certificate signed by each of them. I hugged them all, and cried and sobbed. I am proud and relieved. My chair-mates today are talkative and thrilled for me. We speak about the gift of this and how we've learned to expand time. Each moment is an eternity. There is no guilt. When we are tired, we nap. When hungry, we eat. We are present within our task, wholly there for what we do. My tree outside the window still has no leaves, but the front Zen garden is now complete.

The man next to me, a young one, spoke of how he has always been a private person, and now he trusts his voice and is speaking out. He always read what others had to say, not believing he had anything valuable to add. Now, he sees that he does. He says this experience has been "surreal." He is young and healthy, and, just like that, he had surgery and was in chemo, and it is a gift. He feels he has been resurrected. I understand. I have earned the "Pomp and Circumstance" sung for me today. I am proud of my Certificate of Achievement.

It is time for it to be over, because "we" could not find a place to insert. My veins are worn out and the drip kept stopping, so today was a long infusion day as the needle was moved from one vein to the next. I was calm throughout and found myself saying, "What else would I be doing? What am I rushing toward? All is here. This is enough." And yet, I watched the clock like a hungry hawk does a mouse. I counted minutes, and then seconds. My spring has come!

Yesterday, when I was in my dark night and dark forest of the soul, I read Leo Tolstoy's story, "The Death of Ivan Ilych." Here are some of the last lines that evoke clarity in me:

> *He tries to ask for forgiveness for what he missed in life. The word forgiveness, though, comes out, "Forego." He waved his hand, knowing that He whose understanding mattered would understand.*

> *And suddenly it grew clear to him that what had been oppressing him and would not leave him was all dropping away at once from two sides, from ten sides, and from all sides.*

> *"How good and simple!" he thought. "And the pain?" he asked himself. "What has become of it? Where are you pain?" He turned his attention to it.*

> *"Yes, here it is. Well, what of it? Let the pain be." "And death ....where is it?"*

> *He sought his former accustomed fear of death and did not find it. "Where is it? What death?" There was no fear because there was no death. In place of death there was light.*

> *"So that's what it is!" he suddenly exclaimed aloud. "What joy!"*

> *"Death is finished," he said to himself. "It is no more!"*

Jessica, the nurse practitioner, said even though I am on antibiotics, I can have a glass of wine. Steve took off from work and picked me up from chemo world. We went out to eat, complete.

Evening:

I work on my gifts for those who have cared for me. I return tomorrow for my shot of Neulasta, so I will give gifts then. See's Candy is a given. I work on my card, and then realize I must paint silk hearts. I search for the paints. Though I meant to simplify, and have everything open and available, they are hidden. When I find them, I paint and cut out silk hearts. Energy comes when I'm inspired, and I'm up late into the night. I notice Cat Mandu is aging. I try and prepare, and know I can't. His passing will be another letting go.

March 8:

I wake feeling well, as though chemo has never happened. It feels so over. Of course, I have the shot of Neulasta today, which always throws a noose around me, but it is wonderful to be up, awake and feeling so wonderful, generously full of love, hope and joy.

I receive the shot, and — just like that — I feel bad. It is odd to go from feeling well to not feeling well at all. Each time I hope it will be different, and each time it is the same, and of course, this is the last time.

I check out the drug *Arimidex* online. I am to take it for five years. It shuts off all estrogen, which affects the bones. It is odd to make life decisions based on studies of a few thousand women for a few years, and I am grateful for life. It is hard to take it all seriously, because most of the time I feel fine, except after I go to the doctor. Anyway, my spirits are high, and I am well, and I need a nap.

Are you ready

> *to drop balls like Galileo,*
> *from the Tower of Pisa,*
> *and see that all objects fall to the ground*
> *at the same speed,*
> *except feathers and parachutes,*
> *but that is about friction,*
> *and a very different thing.*

> *Are you ready like Newton to notice*
> *an apple hitting the top of your head, or maybe*
> *not hitting your head, but dropping at your feet,*
> *and then, do you think, hmmmm,*
> *perhaps a law is in effect*
> *and could be defined by me?*

> *Are you ready to paint your heart on silk*

> *and give it away,*
> *to carry out trash and see it recycled*
> *or carried to the dump*
> *and buried and reused*
> *like a parachute*

> *dropping slowly*

> *so a person can land*
> *without straining any muscles*
> *or breaking any bones?*

> *Are you ready*

> *to bow?*

— Cathy

Looking Back: Cathy

I bow in thanks.

Looking Back: Jane

What happens in the long middle distance when the end is still not ready to be gained, when repetition and constant fear has the power to numb or put one to sleep, when doing so could forfeit the end? What Cathy did with the end of chemo in sight, radiation still to come, in the middle of the path between discovery and cure, was to use whatever was there to take the next step and the next: talisman, counting, imagining the change, paying attention to the smallest shift, being here, owning and sharing her particular experience, trusting that others would hear her and value her telling of the story. She had such confidence in this approach and gave herself over to it entirely. It became her life. Sometimes I wondered, maybe even doubted, what part my brief daily presence played.

Looking Back: Cathy

Jane, how could you ever doubt what you gave?

I bow. Namaste!

Kali

March 9:

The sun is out, and Mandu insisted on sleeping on me this morning, keeping me in bed longer that I would ordinarily allow. As I reflected, I felt invisible bandages unwrap from my head. Tears fell as I considered how I went from feeling I would live forever, to thinking I would not live at all. It has been quite a journey. I move my hands over my eye sockets and thank my veins. I am grateful to be here. I am.

I felt called to Rodeo Beach today. The wind was blowing and icy cold. I held onto my wool hat, with my sun hat over it, and trudged along until I found a sheltered place in the rocks. The beach at Rodeo is formed of tiny, smooth colorful rocks. I caressed my fingers with them. The tide was low, and the clouds offshore were in a line, holding hands.

March 10:

I feel pretty well this morning. The week delay in chemo helped me. There is some aching, but not too bad. My mind is fuzzy, so I write an ode to Chemo Brain, Chemo Mind.

Chemo Mind

> *Try to catch it like a butterfly in a net.*
> *It flies and teases,*
> *and plunges in breezes,*
> *until like the sun, it sets.*

— *Cathy*

On Saturday four wild turkeys flew into the garden. Tomorrow snow is forecast below a thousand feet.

It is all the sweet days in between the extraordinary -

Regular and comforting -
Full of, what, I can't remember
Those that leave no mark or stain on tender memory

These are the days that please me.

— Jane

March 11:

Lightning struck outside our bedroom window last night, followed by a thundering crash. The light seemed to strike my dreams. I lived in fairy tales the rest of the night, and then woke to pull out baskets, bunnies, chicks, and eggs for spring.

Elaine sent me Thich Nhat Hahn's words on "fear" the day I was in fear mode. I didn't read them then, but today I hold my feelings and emotions like a bouquet, and lean in to sniff and read the words she sends. He gives steps of welcoming and acceptance to transform the feelings, the fear. I type with Mandu's chin on my arm. He needs my warmth, and I need his.

Jeff and Jan have set their date. They will be married September 10. We've all waited a long time for everything to come together and be just right.

I notice the only thing I have to groom is my expression. There is no hair to comb, no lashes to mascara. I only need to warm a smile.

A friend has been cleared of breast cancer after fighting five years. She is surprised to feel tired now that the battle is over. We put down our fists and let go, feel the waiting fatigue.

I lie down and look up at the ceiling, and am caught on movement and design. It is like a spinning fan. What creates it? I look around the living room, intrigued. Then I realize it is the movement of water in a bowl outside, a bowl filled with specially chosen rocks and a metal

156

dragonfly, now filled with newly fallen water of spring. If water and sun outside can make art on my ceiling, then what else is there when I pause to look and perceive?

I come across a poem by Tess Gallagher called "The Red Devil". The description sounds familiar. Yes, it is the drug they pushed into my veins, the one that would have required a skin graft if it had slipped. Adriamycin! There are reminders of what I've been through. For now, I rest.

March 14:

This morning my thoughts are with my dear friend and comfort, Cat Mandu. He is eating little, though we entice. This morning he was not interested in the milk in my cereal bowl. I asked him to help me get through chemo. He has done that. He often lies on the places in me that hurt. He may still recover, and yet I see him letting go. He has lived over twenty years, and he is not in pain. He sleeps curled in his precious little ball, raises his head when there is a change. He still hops up on the desk, pointing out that he is more important than computer keys and a screen, as of course he is. He is my companion, healer, and friend. He is a brave, true heart. I trust that nature, his nature, knows what to do, and when to part.

I am able to listen to music. The chemo was so discordant in my system, so jarring, that I was unable to take in outside stimulation, but now, I'm beginning to do so. I slowly return to myself. My feet are still. The vibration has stopped. There is no pain.

Some have asked why I didn't use more pain pills. Just as I don't believe in covering up stench with perfume, I haven't wanted to cover up pain with pills. There is a reason for pain, and if I obscure it, I might push beyond what is right for me to do. As much as is reasonably possible, I want to stay present with what is true for me, knowing that pain will eventually change, dissipate. Though the pain was continuous on Sunday, by Monday it began to decrease, and today is fine.

Kali

*Living within
the house of myself
I dance with the tiger's tail
as it swings
from the mouth
of a mouse*

*rainbows offer a curve
for the sky to peruse
the movement of life and death as it shifts
like the wake in a glass*

water holds

then splits.

— Cathy

Rain follows hail.

Tea kettle burns dry.
The lock has seized, refuses keys.
By morning I am a small pile in a scramble of covers.
Your side of the bed has forgotten you.
Through it all, the iris stand fragile, steadfast, blue.

– Jane

Looking Back: Cathy

Kali is a goddess who sings and dances in the presence of mortality, and teaches that a well-lived life is woven not only with joy, but also with sorrow, pain, illness, and death. When we come to accept this, our life is rich.

The drumming beat of chemo was beginning to slow. I knew there was more to go and the light at the end of the tunnel beckoned, vivid and bright.

I attended an Arlo Guthrie concert with my family. It started at three, perfect for me. He said because the world is so troubled right now, we can do something very small and make a difference. The aim is peace, and we each can do our piece.

I am able to do more and more each day, appreciate each part of my life as it returns. There are leaves on the trees, shoes on my feet, and the iris are in bloom.

Looking Back: Jane

During those days in March, I was in a place of loss. Patterns and connections I'd been relying on were falling apart. I was filled with sadness about events in my own life. Even though Cathy would tell me that her pain was no different from mine or anyone else's, as it was all just pain, it was hard to share my troubles with Cathy. In my own sadness, it seemed like everything I reached towards moved away from me. The familiar was replaced by the odd and the frightening–the tiger's tail in the mouse's mouth, the night terrors and the monsters of insomnia.

And yet, each morning as we talked and as we wrote, my hope emerged like an iris in the rain, and it was possible to believe again. Cathy was navigating through her illness, picturing her health. I began to be with what was happening for me, rather than shielding Cathy or myself from my own difficulties. I began to see that I could feel my own struggle without collapsing into it, too.

160

Enough

March 15:

Chemo moves through in waves, so my feet and legs again feel tingly and numb. I stay with the waves, hear a few drops of rain, and the rest is silence, open as my brain, undefined right now by word or task. When the sun appears it is tentative, as though surprised to touch the land directly without the veil of hail, clouds, or snow.

I watch Mandu eat, and Jeff and I decide to take him to the vet. We learn that he is doing well for a cat of his age and we will allow the natural process to unfold.

The Last Straw

I lose my mother

toss her ashes with the golden light of fairies,
and stay robin's breath cheery
in celebration of the spring of her light and her life.

I have a mammogram, sonogram, biopsy,
lumpectomy and removal of three lymph nodes,
do chemotherapy for four months, through
Thanksgiving,

Christmas, and New Years, and into the spring.

I lose the hair on my head,
pubic hair, eyelashes, eyebrows,
and skin peels off my feet in sheets.

I welcome the lessons and reception of love,

but when my beloved Cat Mandu,
friend and companion
for over twenty years appears to be sick,
I stamp my foot and shout, "That's it! ENOUGH!"

— Cathy

161

The garbage trucks grumble up the hill.

One throaty robin makes good use of the sun.
The old cat eats today.
You have turned yourself inside out.
We both imagine who are children will be.
The monsters under our beds are here for good.
All dreams before the long sleep.

— Jane

I whisper into your ear.

I can't remember your face.
Your voice has melted.
Your eyes, once turned away,
Now look outward and up.
I love you the best.
This is the truth.
I have never told anyone.

— Jane

162

Looking Back: Cathy

Cat Mandu helped carry me through chemo and then radiation, with his presence and attention. Each time I returned from chemo and crawled into bed, he lay upon me, absorbed my pain, and hurt. On the day I sat with him, watching him eat, I hoped my presence would return his gift. My poetic outburst gave us time. We settled in peacefully, and he was here until June.

At this time my eyes were often wet in appreciation of breath, my lungs moist in passing grief.

In the fall when the tree outside the chemo room dropped all its leaves, I appreciated the more spacious view of Mount Tam, the open focus. Now I wanted intensity, the burn of sunlight on paper when channeled through a magnifying glass. I yearned to continue my appreciation of the 'tent of no-thought' as I anchored it with stones. I had reveled in openness, and I wanted focus to return. I was ready for Chemo Mind to move on through. I had had enough.

Looking Back: Jane

For many months, Cathy had allowed me into her life to see how the awareness of the body's tenuousness is apparent in her. She had looked at her life and recognized that it could leave her.

Through her sharing, I now can also more fully imagine a life and world without me, when my body has done all the work it can do. It is that body—that faceless face, that voiceless voice—that our morning writing gave me the perspective to whisper to. This body of mine that I have so long taken for granted has, like a donkey, carried me through life. It is this 'you who I have loved the best' for letting me feel my time on earth. It was a surprising realization to me that I had so rarely acknowledged how amazing it is to be embodied and to be grateful to my own body for that experience.

163

164

Part 3:
March to June

Radiate

March 16:

Each time I type "Good Morning," I feel and think, "Good Mourning." I continue to monitor Mandu's breaths, each day a balance of in and out, sunrise, sunset.

March 17:

It is St. Patrick's Day. All is green and new. When Jane and I talk in the morning, I point out that our focus has been around me, but I am feeling well, so our writing may change. I still have a multitude of medical appointments and 33 times of radiation, but I am coming back to life. Today I feel well enough for some masterful cries.

I had not really understood what was meant about chemo — the "dying and coming back" — but today I do. There is no more chemo for me, no more attempts to be hearty, no more falseness in trying to greet the infusion room with a joke and a smile. I settle into the green of the day with wide open eyes.

St. Patrick's Day

See through green colored glasses
   the renewal of spring
         as light
      milks your gaze
         churning butter
            to rings.

 Swirl laughter in ribbons,
    through you and your guides.

Write notes on clouds with sea urchin spines.

            The needles of Zen
               round simply and glide.

      Place lanterns like leprechauns in yawns of the night.

— Cathy

Everything that's green calls out to me today.

The old dog's house opens its roof to sky.
Slung between trees, the hammock waits for sun.
Lavender, rosemary, sage spill along the wall.

Look, they say, as small as we are
We are here and here and here.
Come to us.

— Jane

Looking Back: Cathy

I was enjoying my reprieve. Leprechauns seemed to dance around me, as angels had once appeared to repair my wounds. I felt well enough to feel sad. It takes energy for sorrow, and now I had energy for sorrow and joy. Discernment was on the return, choice. These were benchmark days, and I clapped for inhalation, exhalation, and the space between. I was grateful to clap, to know there was connection in seizing one moment and tracking it with the next. I also knew that Jane and I had twined like strands in a rope, like DNA, and now we were headed toward a deep waterfall plunge into a pond where we didn't know what would emerge. The time was coming to divide.

I, a caterpillar, reaching out from the edge of a leaf, was spinning on the words of Dylan Thomas, "The force that through the green fuse drives the flower / Drives my green age."

In this, I was aware of the moments, of how we divide the 8,700 hours in a year into moments and fill them with people, events, work, sleep, and play, and yet still, for most of us, there are holes, empty space. Those moments are the ones we have the ability to stretch as easily as those spaces in the hammock that open as we drop in.

Looking Back: Jane

The chemotherapy was done. Cathy was emerging as both herself and as a new self that she had grown in dealing with cancer. As she came back to life, I realized I had allowed the idea of death – my death – into my thoughts each day. How different growing old could be if I could see each new day as a new life entering me, as if through the eyes of a baby, a child; if I could live each morning and afternoon with the energy of the adolescent, the adult; if I could reflect on each evening through my wisdom, and welcome the little death of every night. With death and life so close to me each day, where would the fear be? Would there be room for anything but joy?

In the end, our stories are told by what remains. As Cathy and I wrote together, my mother was packing all her worldly things - giving them away, and selling them - in preparation for her final move. To me she gave the letters she had written and received. Of all the things she could have given me, it was these thoughts and sentiments that she had chosen to give breath to, that meant the most to me.

It is the same for these poems Cathy and I wrote every morning. Having given them voice, they now hold more than their words. They hold the feelings of Cathy's journey and mine, as we walked it day by day as friends.

Patience

March 18:

Though I want to keep believing the chemo has washed through, my feet are tingling. I have twinkle toes. I am twinkle feet. I look up and see the moon. It appears still and yet, soon I see it through the needles of the redwood tree. It twinkles, too.

March 20:

I'm feeling much better, and now I see that when I have more energy than I need to survive, I start judging how I utilize my time. Why do we struggle so to be satisfied, and why do I say *we*, when I mean I?

Patience

Precious the tears and rain

caught on the stream in spring

as it runs with the sky

like a kite on a string

— Cathy

My life is this one day.

I am chasing it with a butterfly net.
My swooping efforts crosshatch air.
Nearly everything slips away.
Most of what I catch is light.
Or has wings bruised and dog-eared by my chase.
Sometimes one needle-bright moment enters.
A girl in braids bites into fresh brown bread.

– Jane

Radiation

March 21:

I see the radiation oncologist, Dr. Halberg. Last time the staph infection was spreading. This time there are blue vases filled with daffodils from the American Cancer Society, and one is for me. The flowers help calm my trepidation. Miserable as chemo was, I knew what it was, knew what to expect. I listen as she again explains the odds. Tomorrow, the machine and I meet, and I have a long appointment to get set up and trained. Until then, I practice breathing in slowly and steadily and holding my breath for fifteen to twenty seconds.

My full energy will not return for a year or two. There will be no low-cut shirts for me as the breast tissue goes all the way up to the collarbone. I learn the routine and how to change into my cotton gown and sit and wait. My feet will continue to bother me, but I am considered lucky because I can sleep at night. Dr. Halberg says, "Although you will be sore and tired, this is not chemo. A person is "in chemo". This is different than that."

March 22:

Today in an op-ed piece in the *New York Times* by Peter Salgo, he says that HMO's give doctors seven minutes with a "customer." He says patients became first 'consumers' and then 'customers' in the medical world.

This hasn't been my experience at Marin Cancer Institute. Dr. Halberg spent at least 45 minutes with me yesterday, answering every type of question and reassuring me. The woman who will work with me today is coming back from her lunch fifteen minutes early so I won't have to make two trips up, and can fit in both medical appointments I need today. I realize that this isn't the experience of many or most in this country right now.

The CT/simulator took a long time and was strange. I felt like I was in a science fiction movie, watching a Pac Man to know when to breathe and when to hold my breath. There were palm trees painted on the ceiling and Hawaiian music to boost relaxation.

I decide it is time to shop, since I'm told I'll need to wear camisoles, not bras. In the dressing room, I see the back of my head and how huge it is without hair. I never realized how much room there is back there. I try to imagine hair. I discover that most tops are cut below the collar bone. I am being radiated in a larger area than most. I also learn that lanolin smells like sheep. I hope I get used to the smell. I walk past a place offering a discount on laser hair removal. I can only shake my hairless head at the goofiness of this marvelous world.

March 23:

In the shower I see my red 'Sparkie' marks, a bloody splash on my right, odd symbols on the left, and a third eye on the sternum. I receive my radiation registration tattoos next Thursday. These will be my first tattoos.

If I choose, I can have my right breast "raised" to match the left, since radiation makes the one radiated "perkier." I choose not to. Two breasts, with one reaching toward the ground, and the other toward the sky, will remind me of the balance I am trying to attain and retain in my life.

I learn that my heart doesn't drop when I lie on my back, so my appointment time is changed to accommodate a different machine, the newer, more modern one.

Calvin Trillin has a beautiful tribute to his wife Alice in the *New Yorker* this week. Radiation gave her twenty-five extra years of life, and yet, when she died, the doctor said "her heart had been destroyed by radiation." I see how I am choosing to ignore the long-term side effects in all of this. If I gain twenty-five quality years, how can I be anything less than thrilled? If I only gain five years, I will be thrilled. One year. Two! A minute! Please!

March 24:

I'm reading books on travel, nurturing a need for wider boundaries than the last six months have provided. A coyote appears in Central Park. I wonder if that is how the first cancer cell feels, undomesticated, wild, alone.

I receive a card from my brother with Tibetan monks speeding downhill on a roller coaster, their arms up in the air. My brother writes, "SMILE!!! You're on the DOWNHILL RUN!!"

Ode to Eyelashes

taken for granted
until chemo removes them
lash by lash, upper and lower
slowly thinning
until one day they are gone.

Eyes gaze as puddles, bare
no grasses surrounding
the wake of the pond.

The lashes
of the whip
are gone, too
only kindness
for what comes along,
no filtered flogging of the view.

I think of dew.

— Cathy

Heat changes everything.

The day of one who picks tomatoes slows.
Steel turns to butter.
Long ago the heat brought sorrows.

It drowned the orchard in its light.
And yet I did not know how much I loved you until the
onions melted.

– Jane

Looking Back: Cathy

Without eyelashes, my eyes were huge, unblocked. Other than applying mascara and using an eyelash curler for special occasions, I had paid little attention to my eyelashes; now they were gone. The open gaze stirred something in me and I found acceptance, and a new ability to receive. Charlotte Selver used to talk about people using their eyes like forks. The knife and fork of dissection and judgment were gone, replaced with a new ingestion of ease.

I like to run my fingers around the socket of the eye, the seven bones that meet to form the orbit, feel how huge that space is, and bring in the world with that immensity without any need to censor or squint.

I did learn that eyelashes have a purpose other than beauty. They keep out dust and yet I was grateful for no filters as I looked forward to what radiation would bring.

Looking Back: Jane

As the time for my vacation neared, I felt guilty about leaving Cathy without our morning calls for support. Even though I had entertained occasional doubts that my morning calls provided any significant encouragement at all, guilt was with me. I tried to imagine the heat and burn of radiation. I tried to think about what Cathy might experience while I was gone. I wondered if there were things I could do before I left, and while I was gone.

But something shifted in me when Cathy read her poem about the loss of her eyelashes. I experienced through Cathy's acceptance of the way things were for her, a renewed sense of what kindness to my own self might look like. I sat with that. With some practice I found I was able to hold both feelings - the guilt I felt about leaving while she was still dealing with illness and treatment, and my excitement and anticipation for my trip - without negating either feeling.

Watching the Breath

March 26:

My niece Katy informs me that she is going to be a butterfly in her ballet recital. She says, "I love being a butterfly. Our play is called *The Four Seasons*. I'm the transition from spring to summer."

I'm currently the transition from winter to spring, and soon, I'll be the transition from spring to summer. I've never seen it so clearly before.

March 28:

I am with the breath, as I practice for my time with the radiation machine. I breathe in evenly, and hold my breath so that my heart drops and is not radiated along with the breast.

I have three medical visits today to ensure I begin radiation on Thursday.

There was a woman at radiation today, a young, pretty one, with just the softest coating of hair on her head. I later learned her name was Kate, Kate Behr. She said it was her first day out without her scarf and she felt naked. She had only four chemo treatments, instead of my eight, and her last one was January 3, so I was disappointed to see how long the hair takes to grow back. I had my last chemo treatment on March 7, so if I am on her schedule, I won't begin to get hair until June. I am disappointed, but then I have to laugh. Before, I was content to live. Now, I want to live *and* have hair. I find it funny.

I realized today when I looked into Kate's eyes, and she looked into mine, that those of us who are so obviously 'in' it, never smile at each other. It is like the communication is on a different level. It is the strangest thing, and it isn't with everyone, but I have caught it with some. It is like we are taking each other in whole, caught and swimming in each other's eyes, where there is no trace of, or need for, a smile. Perhaps it is how babies and young children look at each other. There is recognition. It is a moment, and a moment is all there ever is, and it is so clear when one truly meets another, both standing as magnifying glass and mirror.

Rich Breath, Rich Life

Breath

a bucket I fill to make sand castles

to lift

and texture the beach.

Fairy homes

wash in and out

cleanse

in the life of the sea.

I toss a rope to the moon

match the tides inside

leash on currents

like pollen and seeds.

I dance with bees.

— Cathy

We were on a family car trip through the redwoods.

The motel pool was blue and cold.

I raced my brother, jumped feet first into the deep end.

I was breathless when my toes touched bottom.

Through the dimpled chlorine surface, far above, my father stood.
His back was turned.
He didn't see me, couldn't save me.
Heart held my breath to surface.
I never told them I'd almost drowned.

— Jane

Looking Back: Cathy

Elizabeth Barrett Browning said, *"He lives most life whoever breathes most air."* I was with the quality of the breath, the texture and how it formed and moved, like waves in the sea. I used the breath like sand to cleanse. I went under with it, and popped back up again and again. Perhaps this is what we always do, and some moments are more noticeable and memorable than others. And yet, I know we also need to cultivate the pause, to kick off the bottom of our thoughts, and rise anew again. I felt tied to currents and tides, alive with the spread of life like pollen and seeds, and awake to the curious dance of bees.

Since air was my playground, both inside and out, how free could I be as I guided my breath to the commands that radiation demands? I was aware of protecting my heart and wanting to do everything exactly right. I tossed a rope to tie my breath to the moon.

Looking Back: Jane

The poem Cathy wrote in which she practiced the special breathing needed to protect her heart through radiation, comforted me. I could see her toss a rope to circle the moon and tie it firmly to her heart and breath. I could keep that image with me as I traveled. No matter where I was, I could see the moon and know it was helping her breathe correctly for radiation. As she took care of herself, she also took care of me. I knew she would have powerful aides to be by her side while I was gone. I let that in.

More Radiation Set-Up

March 30:

Jane leaves for Spain tomorrow, and is very busy, but we make time to talk, and then I write alone. I realize how sad I am this morning because I don't really like the radiation place. Oddly enough, I am looking back on the chemo room as a place of some delight. I had my place, my chair. I knew how to prepare.

I am frightened of radiation world, where I sit in a room with other people in thin, cotton robes, so many people very thin, some with no hair, and I am not so fond of machines, either. I'm sure I will get used to it, but I am not there yet.

So today after all that anticipation about crowding and people in robes and such, I walk into the radiation waiting room, and there is no one there but me. I am called in and introduced to the four computers that will monitor me. I lie down and three people work with my placement. There are water lilies on the ceiling. I listen to Chopin. Pictures are taken, and the doctor is called in and more pictures are taken. Chopin is getting excited, and I can barely hear the voice instructing me when to breathe and when to hold my breath. Chopin is exuberant. It is hard not to match my breath to his, but I try to keep it just the same. I am told when I have not inhaled enough air, or when there is too much. It is hard to find a natural breath with all this scrutiny, but I do. I am tattooed, four pin-pricks, and I am done.

Elaine came to my home yesterday. It was our first meeting in person, our first physical touch. She gave me a smoky-quartz stone with rainbows for healing. I met her through technology, the internet, and that has been our connector, especially in the night as she healed from brain surgery, and I dealt with chemotherapy. Now we touch and talk and paint our hearts on silk in circular frames. She takes home a gift, a Sacred Hoop, her painting, her heart, on silk.

Chemo mind

I lost it slowly
   never noticed the steps disappearing
   until clouds, sea, sky, and I were one

   Now, the steps come back

   I stand on each, look around,
      struggle to remember
      the names of trees
      and how leaves come forth
         and fall —

      I know where bumblebees go when it rains
         how they cohere and hug
            buzz and bond —
         The winged drapes strengthen the hive.

            Home, home, rise and sink
               Revive with tides

— Cathy

181

Looking Back: Cathy

I continued to learn how ridiculous it was to anticipate and dread. I was uncomfortable with what I perceived as the chaos of radiation the first time I went, but when I returned, the waiting room was empty, and I sat alone in silence and peace. It said everything about the waste involved in expectation and worry. Am I finished learning yet?

Looking Back: Jane

Cathy's poem on March 30th was my first 'aha' about the effects that chemo had had on her mind and thinking. I'd felt a softness, an acceptance in Cathy during her chemo treatments, but I'd attributed it more to the slowing-down process of illness, and the slowing down that Cathy had practiced. I hadn't attributed her acceptance to the effects of those chemicals that ran through her blood, throughout her system and her brain. I had found a memory of being at the bottom of a swimming pool, out of breath, that helped me experience the feeling of knowing there is gap or distance between myself and others. The wonder for me is that even while she was inside that gap, she was able to give the experience words.

March 30:

Jane plants a poem for me as she leaves for Spain.

He traveled in a business suit by train.

By day he would sit in the vista cruiser.
From his briefcase he'd pull out white bread sandwiches and eat.
The bones of the world slid past, past, past him.
On a yellow legal pad he would write as fast as he saw.
At night he would get out at the first station after dark.
He'd find a diner, eat some soup.
Then he'd staple some of his yellow sheets of paper to phone
*   poles.*
Before dawn, he would sleep, sitting up in the train station.
He'd take the first train out
Leaving his poems to flutter like bandages in the wind.

– Jane

Looking Back: Cathy

I was excited that Jane was going to Spain. She had been loyal and faithful, so I was grateful she would have a break. We were so connected at this point, that I felt I was traveling with her, too. We were two particles that, once together, even when pulled apart, respond to the spin of the other. We were bound and buoyed. Her poems were "bandages on the wind."

Looking Back: Jane

As I left for Spain, the doubts I'd had that writing together would be enough, or offer enough support, returned...but in a new way. If it really was meaningful, how could I be leaving?

Looking Back: Cathy

Of course our time together was meaningful and how could you not enjoy some time away?

We come together and divide, like sand washed by waves, then left to dry. Sometimes sand dries and mounds and sometimes it blows away.

First Day of Radiation

March 31:

Jane is on her way to Spain, and I HAVE HAIR!! Some might call it fuzz, but I can see it without a magnifying glass and I feel it. My hair's return is a sign of health. My hair has survived, as have I.

When I arrive for radiation, there is a new jigsaw puzzle on the table, and rain sparkles in the garden. The trees are beginning to get leaves, just like me. We're on the same schedule.

I was scared at first, as this was the first real radiation day, the set-up is so precise, and the breathing is so important, but I was told I did "great." I held my breath the whole 36 seconds, and it was only four times, two in one place, and two in another. The whole thing took about 30 minutes. I have one radiation down and thirty-two more to go.

When I went into the dressing room to change back into my clothes, Shelley, also in a wool cap, introduced herself and told me about the support group, which I have had no energy for, and then introduced me to Diane Brandon, who signed me up for eight Fridays of "Equine Therapy." When I found out about chemo, the only thing that seemed palatable was the possibility of horse therapy. Now, I receive my reward. Jane leaves and something steps in to take her place.

Today a clothing catalog arrives with a "mature" model on the cover. Her hair is short and white, and she is lovely, I'm grateful to note.

April 3:

The rain is soft today and ripens the green. I leave early enough to walk between showers. I feel pretty well, until I think of radiation. I find it nerve-wracking to hold such precise control over my breath. I've studied the breath for years, reaching for the unconscious swing, and now I consciously inhale and hold. Never has it mattered so much that I do it just right.

185

April 4:

My radiation appointment is early, and I still rise early enough to squeeze in a walk beforehand. When I arrive, I'm the first one there and the robes are still warm. Francine, my doctor, is thrilled with the pictures, and how well the machine and I are working together. She says that in two months I won't need a hat and will look "tres chic." Steve thinks I look "tres chic" already, but he is biased.

April 5:

Between the rain and excitement about feeling better as chemo continues to wash on through, I could barely sleep. I was awake much of the night, savoring and welcoming my body back to life.

Today I attended a "Look Good...Feel Better" workshop hosted by the American Cancer Society. We gathered to learn about chemo, radiation, wigs, scarves, turbans, and hats. I was the model, so I got instant feedback. I am a turban/scarf/hat person. Wigs are not for me, though there is a room full of them, and they are free.

Radiation went easily for me today, though the place was in a mess. Both machines broke down today, so everything was behind schedule. People talked as they waited. Though I've been assigned to the newest, most modern machine, I learn that it will still radiate a bit of my heart. One woman comes up from Palm Springs for this machine because Marin Cancer Institute is one of the few places that have one. Also she said these are the best doctors around in the breast cancer field. It's good to have those from afar to remind us how good it is where we are.

The door to the meditation garden was open today, and a lovely breeze wafted in. Someone had placed a bunch of azalea plants in the garden, so it bloomed in pink, rose, and white, and a perky green parrot perched there, too. The sun is shining through the trees, and there are some fluffy, white clouds. Tomorrow I'll have three appointments in the same place. Jane sends a poem from Spain.

Our room is blue.

> *The towels are as big as sails*

> *Alone in the shower the hotel soap remembers some deep sadness.*

> *In the afternoon we sat in the peace of Plaza Sant Neri.*

> *The school there was closed*

> *The restaurant not yet open.*

> *Two plane trees had found their way*

> *Straight as arrows above the buildings*

> *Whose walls were silently healing from the holes of countless executions.*

> *Forever and ever.*

– Jane

Looking Back: Cathy

I lived like a child — cared for and enchanted. All seemed new. I continue even now to meet people who speak of the gift cancer can be. It is so hard to explain the magic of those days, even amidst, or perhaps because of the parts that were tough. What I believe now though is that we share each part and unite the joy, anger, sorrow, fear. I was a focal point, carrying a great many into the circle of my care. I was the center of the carousel — the love and healing intention of professionals, family, and friends circling around.

Looking Back: Jane

It was almost Easter. The flower shops in Barcelona were full of palms and lilies, and the lottery tickets bore the face of Christ. Cathy had begun radiation, and I was sitting in the farmer's market in Barcelona with Spanish workmen who were having breakfasts of olives, beer, and ham. Behind me, a young woman minding a fish stall was humming a pining love song with the radio. In front of me in the open air, the barman was making me a Spanish tortilla thick with eggplant, zucchini, and potatoes. How can this be my life when a good friend is struggling with illness?

Later, on our way to Granada, I read *Tales of the Alhambra*. I used Washington Irving's words to imagine the Alhambra before we got there. The reality was so much more than I could ever have imagined, and I remember hoping: "That's what recovery will be for Cathy - a life better than she remembers, better than what she can imagine right now." That night in our hotel, in the tiny bathroom, I found a comb wrapped in plastic. I mailed it to Cathy to help her imagine her new hair.

Changing Focus

April 6:

Radiation went well, as did my bone scan. I now have only 28 more radiations to go, though I'm trying not to count. Part of me wants to just let them happen as they do, and another part knows it is probably important to remember how many there are to go. Today, I felt the radiation as it hit. Perhaps, I'm becoming more sensitive, or I'm paying more attention. The music today was Benny Goodman, and again, it was hard to stay still and not tap my toes.

April 7:

My breast is turning pink and is a bit sunburned. I have radiation again today, and then my first experience with the horses. This is exciting and new. Cindy Cantril, who heads the Marin Cancer Institute Resource and Recovery Center, has been instrumental in developing the Healing with Horses Equine Therapy program for people recovering from cancer in Marin. This day opens like a parasol with multi-colored rays.

I arrive at radiation early, so I have time to walk along the marsh and observe the ducks. The jigsaw puzzle is out and only needs twenty pieces to complete. And who completes it? I do! A photo is taken of the completed puzzle and I get to choose the next one. I pick "Water Maidens" and begin. I learn that many people stay an hour or two after their radiation treatment and work with the puzzle. I sneered at the puzzle table when I first saw it, as well as at the attempts to entertain us as though we were children, but now I see it as a gauge. Now I can discern and find form in space. I match the pieces and see colors and shapes differently than before. Specificity and focus return, and the open space of Chemo Mind closes down a bit each day. I'm grateful to find the balance of the two and find focus in space.

It is amazing what passes as an accomplishment for me these days. I am pleased to have finished the puzzle and begun another. Steve has been in NY, and I could see that when I told him I finished the puzzle and got to choose the next one, he didn't understand how something so small could seem so important. And yet, for me, it is a tangible step. I gather those steps like flowers in my hands; only I can make a bouquet.

In this short time, I am comfortable with radiation world. Everyone is friendly. I'm gaining a new appreciation of machinery. It seems the physicist is always at Marin Cancer Care to care for the machines. He loves them, and I am getting comfortable with mine.

A new person is trained today, so the breath part is more challenging. She isn't as quick on the part where I get to breathe, but she will get there. Anna and I had developed a rhythm and I appreciate her ability to sense what I need and can do.

The nurse today makes it clear that this weekend is to be about resting. After radiation, I enjoy a break, and then drive out to Marin Stables in Fairfax for the first session of equine therapy for cancer patients and survivors. Jim McDermott, who heads the program, makes it clear that we should come rested. Since I tire so easily, that is a tall order. He says continuously that we are to "rest before we are tired, eat before we are hungry, and drink before we are thirsty." I need the constant reminder; it is easy to forget. We enjoy the food and drinks prepared by an army of excited volunteers. Everything we need is here. The message is self-care.

We sit in a circle and meet each other, our mentors, and the horses. We humans take turns being horse and rider. We learn to be in the moment, like a horse, to guide and respond to the energy of another, and to use our own.

When I leave the stables and pass the tall trees at Samuel P. Taylor Park, they seem like wands waving over me, telling me to sleep. I am Dorothy in the poppy fields in the Wizard of Oz. I am tired and fulfilled, and grateful to go home and sleep. As much as I love it, this is a push for me, and I am thrilled to be part of this group.

April 8:

I stopped in Point Reyes Station yesterday before equine therapy, bought a book by Alice Hoffman, and learned that she is a cancer survivor. Why am I so irritated by these words, 'cancer survivor'? I thought to survive you had to do something. All I did was show up. I went to appointments and made decisions. Can I pat myself on the back? Maybe! Do I want it on my resume? Not yet! Perhaps it is that I can't take in what has happened and what I have done. Perhaps, in some way, I still don't believe this has happened to me.

At radiation world, I hear families talk as they gather in the waiting rooms. It's an odd place, and with all the attempts at cheeriness and calm, there is an undercurrent of fear and sometimes, pain. Some people bring someone with them, so there are usually others in the inner waiting room besides the patients, even though only the patients themselves are supposed to be there. The older couples often sit close together as a unit of one. One man is trying to decide whether to do chemo, and whether to give his long, silver-gray ponytail to Locks for Love. Despite the discussion, he doesn't seem to grasp that he will lose all his hair. I see it is hard for men to lose their hair, too. Two elderly wives wait for their husbands, oblivious that they are supposed to be in the outer room, and they talk about what their husbands have been through. They're so glad their husbands don't have to do chemo. Two of us sit there with no hair. What is there to say? We've become so androgynous, invisible at times, aware. Tears come.

Finishing the puzzle yesterday was huge for me, because I had a chance to feel genuine joy in the waiting room. I struggle there, despite the garden, flowers, fish, and pictures. Yet, yesterday, I smiled, and so did everyone else. We shared a ritual. A photo of the completed puzzle is in "the completed puzzle book." We paused together for a moment, and then everything and everyone continued on.

After spending time with Jim, the mentors, and the horses, when I picked up the kitchen and the rest of the house, I noticed where my eyes were going, how they move in and out between particular and open focus. For me, chemo mind is open focus, taking things in whole, doing so with no energy, need, or attempt to dissect or judge. It is like being a child. Now I telescope in and out; I have choice. I also know the place between and I live there, too, glimpsing where the pollen globes roam.

I use the word 'between' and now I wonder what it means. Between is separation *or* connection. I am reminded of words I wrote when I came to Rosen: "As much as you may feel a preference for flow, please note at times the edge which evolution probes."

April 10:

When I come to radiation world today, only the outline of a new puzzle is in place on the waiting room table. I'm too tired to fill it in, or care.

I begin to see that The California Cancer Care Center at 1350 South Eliseo in Greenbrae is about community. People strive to

191

understand and bring hope to pain. There's a new artwork display. The azaleas are gone from the meditation garden. I prefer the simplicity of just the garden, the lines of stones and plants. I learn that the azaleas were decorations for a party to welcome a new machine. This one is a little guy — portable, and about four feet tall.

My machine is mighty and massive. It has a huge eye that blinks. To me, it represents the left brain side of the modern cancer world, the logical and rational. The hugs, touch, and intuitive knowing of horse therapy balance the trust we've placed in technology, precision, and percentages. My health depends on both.

Today is a picture day, so it takes some time. I'm radiated on one side while bare, and then again with what feels like a wet jellyfish flopped across my chest to flatten it. Then, the big eye of the machine moves around and I'm radiated from the other side, both bare and flattened. The novelty has worn off and I am tired of this. This is my seventh day, a day of rest, and though I have had two days of weekend rest, I am tired and depressed.

When I finish, I'm told to wait to see the Social Services person. Why would I need social services? I'm angry, and glad the garden is wet. It fits my mood. I want a life outside this place. Then Sandy, the Social Services person who is also a therapist, appears and leads me to her room. If I had seen her Friday, I would have said all was well, but today, all is not well. I'm angry. I want to feel well. I want hair. I don't want to be here.

Sandy's great, though. She's led support groups for cancer patients for years. She understands when I tell her I want to do cancer *well*. I want my 'normal' life. I'm trying to do what I did before, and I have these appointments, and I can't do them all, and I feel sad. She helps me understand that I'm still *in it* and will be for a long, long time, that I won't feel truly well for a long time. It doesn't just end, she says, and emphasizes over and over again that I didn't cause this, but I also can't prevent it. It's the luck of the draw. I need to understand. I sit with that. Okay, I didn't cause this, and I can't prevent it. This is the luck of the draw. This is the luck of the draw. Humph!! Do I feel better because of that? I'm not sure, but I do see that it is about accepting and letting go.

Sandy says people expect some great transformation with cancer. They want to emerge transformed. Yep, that is I. People think they are going to be different, but the bills still need to be paid, the house still needs to be cleaned, and the food needs to be brought in. Maybe that's what I face; I've put things off. I can't face my taxes and am filing for an

192

extension. But, I also realize I *have* kept things up, and have navigated both the 'real' world and the spacey, scary medical one. How I feel is normal. That's why they have a therapist on staff, and it is amazing that today was my day to see her. I know I'll return to her, and I leave with my assignment, which is to be kind to myself. Okay! That's a tough assignment. Be kind to myself. Why is that so hard? Be kind!!

I am touched by Sandy and her probing and comments. She said I worry the cancer will come back. I hadn't actually thought I was thinking of that, but perhaps I was, because I am glad she said it. She's blunt about how crummy this is. I don't let myself feel it very often. I usually look at what I have gained from it, but today, I hit some wall of exhaustion and I came home and couldn't do anything this afternoon.

Mandu got sick when I had my last chemo treatment. I think he wears down with me, but today he is doing better. He wants me to know that he is a better companion than a horse. I fell asleep with him on my lap and we share a good, warm nap.

April 11:

I feel better today. Something released yesterday in talking with Sandy. I was carrying a heaviness of expectation, and I let that go, renewing myself with sleep.

My hair is growing. At first it was peach fuzz, and now, it's a little more, though it doesn't really show up, because it is so light in color. Still, I can feel it, and I see it in certain light. I am starting to feel a little warmer, so I think it is doing the job it is intended to do.

Today is treatment number eight for me, with only twenty-five to go after today. Today was easy. They had to take pictures again, but it all zipped along. They mixed up the order of patients, so I didn't even have to wait. It was funny, though, because knowing all was well with me, I figured I could speed through, but Francine became interested in my Easter dinner. We are both having honey baked ham from Costco, with sweet Parker House or Hawaiian rolls, and Mendocino hot and sweet mustard. I enjoyed connecting with Francine, who was thrilled that I see radiation as a sideline in my life, not as my actual life. It is definitely a side dish and not the whole meal.

April 12:

Following tradition, the person whose last treatment was today brought cookies to the radiation waiting room. Yesterday, someone brought champagne for their last one. Luckily, they had the last appointment of the day. I like the idea of sharing sparkly, but not before my precise line-up is complete.

I noticed a new painting today, a little one with this quote by Isabel Allende next to it: "....she is lost in the labyrinth of reason and all her security now lies in affection and love."

April 13:

Yesterday I left the machine to immediately enter another room to be given a massage by a man who is legally blind. He has a seeing-eye dog, because he only sees forms and emotions. He used to be a baker. He was part of my treatment yesterday, a lesson in touch, and a lesson in seeing. Marin Cancer Care is clear in their healing treatment. They use machines and they use touch. They want us aware and active in our own healing. They use love and care. Today I expose my new hair to the air, and hang clothes outside to dry. I balance my increasing energy. I let the radio blare 60's music. I am content to notice what I am experiencing and what I need. I am a seed with hair, ready to fly.

April 14:

Each year Good Friday feels like a special day to me. No matter what our beliefs, it feels important to honor dying and resurrection. It feels especially precious this year.

My eyelashes are growing back. Someone asks me what Taxol was like. From this end of the tunnel, it all seems like fairy dust and light. How quickly we forget, or do we? Where are these memories held?

It has been a full day. I've had radiation, more drawing on me, and more pictures. I have had pictures four days this week. I am still not relaxed around the breathing. I am worn out from trying to do it 'just right.' It is odd to have to perform what should be natural. Today, I feel how tiring it is to run up to the cancer institute five times in a week, and breathe just right, have pictures taken, and have radiation sprayed on me. Today is also session two of horse therapy.

Through the horse, I feel my fatigue, and yet I keep going. I do not honor self-care, even though we are continuously told to "Drink before we are thirsty, eat before we are hungry, and rest before we are tired." Next time I will be more aware.

Today we groomed the horses. We began with our hands to get to know the horse and to let the horse know us. Then we used the brush. We worked with 'our' horse to have it step back, go in a circle, and come toward us. We did this through body language. We don't speak. The idea is to communicate telepathically, as horses do.

It is clear that, as a woman of my generation, my body language is submissive. I am here to learn that it is empowering to be dominant through my body language with a 1200-pound animal. The horse wants me to take charge. Horses are prey animals. We are predators. They expect us to be in charge and to know what to do. Though I love to stand and hug Challenger, I also know I can direct him forward and back and in circles through my body language. I learn I have influence over my environment. The horse is a mirror. I see a license plate holder today that says, "Save a horse. Ride a cowboy." These days, I choose a horse. The cowboy will have to wait.

Looking Back: Cathy

I look back and see a time of changing moods. I had the energy to sign up for equine therapy, yet I also felt pushed beyond my very limited reserves. I used the experience as a carrot to pull me further along than was comfortable, and as a spur to get me back on track.

The purpose of horse therapy is to empower, to re-integrate mind and body, and to re-teach natural and intuitive movement and response. We were being instructed as "horse whisperers," to counteract the influence of rules, schedules, and machines.

At the time, I was too exhausted to fully appreciate it. I stumbled along with gratitude and a smile, fatigue being my constant companion. I struggled to believe that all these volunteers chose and felt privileged to be with us. Just by being, we were somehow seen as profound. What a lesson to absorb after all those years of *trying* to be interesting and entertaining. I, like a fish unable to discern water, was unable to understand our appeal. The natural tendency of a sick animal is to hide, yet we were celebrated. That said, I was one of the few still in treatment, and I might have better understood the full impact of the course if I had been out of treatment. It is only now that I can begin to fully absorb the gift.

Looking Back: Jane

From Palm Sunday through Easter Sunday, I was in Sevilla. This is a week called *Semana Santa*, during which the parishioners of every church in town organize a ritual that includes carrying each church's most prized icons – their Madonnas and their tableaus of the Passion of Christ – through the streets to Sevilla's main cathedral. Everyone, young and old, native and non-native, politely crowds the narrow streets each day from afternoon till midnight as the huge floats, carried on the backs of young men, wind their way for miles from their home churches to the town's central cathedral and back again. Blocks of parishioners/penitents, carrying four-foot candles, accompany each float. Most are escorted by bands of drums and bugles.

What struck me most about being there as an outsider, was that I didn't feel like an outsider. It was a community experience. Although the event is Catholic, in another way it seems to belong to the people, not to the church. It's the parishioners of the Sevilla's churches who plan and carry out the event, not the clergy. To me, that imbued the week with the feeling that all of Sevilla, all of Spain, really, took time every year to tell each other stories of human suffering and hope. By the end of the week, it seemed to me, that all human hearts in the city of Sevilla beat together to the drum, and all human ears leaned into the bugles' fading wail.

It was a feeling that in a very subtle way connected me to Cathy. By telling her own story as it happened, by being present for her illness, and by finding ways to imagine her own recovery and well-being, she, like the Sevillians, reminded me that we all have the ability to affect our own lives for the better. Yes, it is true. Churches and religions can provide us with inspiration, and doctors, nurses, hospitals, and treatment can help our bodies heal. But we as people can also provide ourselves and one another with hope. We can support the human desire for basic goodness in each other. We can tell each other stories that inspire all of us to survive and flourish in spite of, and side by side with, all else that happens in our lives.

Easter

April 16:

I went out for a walk and saw the Easter Bunny standing near the fire station. He asked me if I wanted a hug, and I did. A bunny hug! What a day! My family came to visit and play.

April 17:

I lie down for radiation and feel how tired I am when I am there. I want to sleep. Steve says my poems of late don't seem to be in my usual flow. I can't find my flow with so much intrusiveness. I am meant to have blood drawn today, but when I go, they can't find a vein, so I have to return after drinking gallons of water because my veins have decided to hide. My veins and I are tired of being prodded and poked. I don't like having a "standing order" at the lab.

April 18:

Today Dr. Halberg comments on the difference in my speech patterns. She said that when I first came to her, it was clearly an effort for me to speak. I had no energy for words. Now I do. She also said I have more color each time I come. I am grateful for that. She also likes my new blue hat. I learn I am a deep breather. I breathe in fully and savor my exhales. A new person guides me today, and she honors my need for full exhalation, before she guides me again to inhale.

I am feeling layers in myself from working with the horses. I am dreaming of them and their depths. I love their huge eyes and hearts. My heart grows in response, as do my lungs.

April 19:

Today is radiation number fourteen. Though my breast is sore, my morning walk takes me further in the same amount of time. Before I enter the building, I am now able to make it to the top of the hill for a view of the bay.

Each time I go to radiation it seems to take more adjustment time. I have to be placed exactly as I was in the simulation. They measure and adjust, and measure and adjust again. All must be perfect. I breathe and let go, breathe and hold, and then let go. The adjustment is taking longer because I have changed. I have straightened and expanded. I came to radiation tightly held and heavily armored to fend off the next attack. I measured each word and step. Now, this time with the horses is allowing me to return to a natural bubbling. I gain strength and trust.

More pictures are taken of me today. I feel like a super-model. When I leave, a group of people are excitedly analyzing my pictures. I find it funny. I have lived as modestly and invisibly as possible, and now, even my X-rays are the subject of interest to many.

I am pulled out of myself, a flower opened by sun. My cocoon dissolves and there is joy in knowing a wider surround.

April 20:

Today when I arrive, I notice a huge sign proclaiming, "Marin Cancer Institute." There is a new speed bump as I leave. Perfect! It feels just right to have my teeth jarred out of my head as I leave the Marin Cancer Institute. Bah, Humbug, I say. I do not like this place, and yet, of course, I do.

When I comment on the pain, the medical staff informs me I'm halfway through this part. There are twenty-seven of what I am currently having: long radiation from two sides, both exposed, and then, flattened with the rubber jellyfish. The last six will be intense focus in one spot. I guess I am supposed to be excited I'm halfway through this part, but what I'm feeling is pain and fatigue, and concern about the last six. I want to hide.

This was my day for Sandy, the therapist. My breast hurts and I am tired and sleep-deprived. I want to wake naturally, instead of hurrying to get up to radiation. I reach my limits so easily now. My reserves are nil. "Natural," she says. "You're still not recovered from chemo. This will take a year. Be kind to yourself." Ah, yes, those words come back again. Be kind to yourself. I drive home, feeling lighter.

I continue to read about Arimidex. Is it right for me? My hair continues to return. I don't have to shave my legs, but my pubic hair begins. I am eleven again.

April 21:

Yesterday, Elaine suggested that American Ginseng is good for radiation fatigue. I had one cup of tea around five yesterday, and I felt calm and energized. I woke this morning feeling like a million bucks, ready for my day, so now I have American Ginseng in capsule and tea form. Even if it's psychological, it works. Maybe it will get me over the radiation fatigue hump. My breast feels better, so perhaps the pain is connected to fatigue. Today in our third session with the horses, we worked with adapting to the horse, as the horse adapts to us. It is a continual exchange. One woman said she wanted everything to be black and white, always the same, but that is not how this is. Each interaction is new, like life.

The body language with the horses is: Ask, Suggest, Inspire. 'Inspire' is the most forceful. You bring the energy up in your own body, raise it up, and inspire the horse with your energy. If you want the horse to back up, you allow your energy to back up. When the horse follows a suggestion, you release. Human and horse return to neutral again. This is a way to work consciously with our energy and receive instant feedback from the horse.

We need to be clear in ourselves and know what we want to convey to the horse. Horses are telepathic. When I knew what I wanted, and was clear in myself, the horse knew, and responded quickly and correctly. Horses want to please, and they have considerations of their own. They don't like to waste energy. Young ones may, but older ones know how to conserve their energy so they are ready to run when there is a threat. We can learn from horses to live in neutral, unless there is a need to mobilize our energy for response.

If we become frightened on a horse, and wave our arms and kick and shout for the horse to stop, what happens? The horse responds to our raised, frightened energy and goes faster. Instead, pause. Convey to the horse it is time to stop. We practice the pause. Inhale. Pause. Exhale. Pause. Ah!

The horses give instant feedback as to whether we are present with ourselves. It is humbling to see how often my mind wanders. When it goes, so does the horse. I worked with Challenger, and then another person worked with Challenger. While I saw Challenger as gentle, she saw him as tough and difficult. Our mentor said we see what we are. We are given feedback on perception and projection. She said because I am gentle, I see gentleness in my horse. I certainly fall in love with my horse each time we meet, and feel my heart grow horse huge. I love to hug, kiss, and pat my horse. Horse therapy works for me.

April 22:

Mandu and I are thrilled that it's Saturday and I don't have to rush to radiation. Mandu grooms himself and continues to point out to me that he has almost all the advantages of a horse, and is better packaged for both size and ease of care.

I woke this morning in the radiation position, my body slightly skewed, and my left arm overhead. I am hoping my body/mind interprets that as a healing position, and I am healing in my sleep.

I participate in a painting class today, one that is offered for those who are in, or have been in, breast cancer treatment. I enjoy the music and the chance to feel where my arm and hand want to go. I like my paintings, as well as the joy and relaxation they represent. I think of Bali, where living is art and all is worship. I wish that notion lived and thrived more obviously and clearly here. We are so divided into work and play.

Cancer was an obvious subject of discussion as we painted. I'm still struggling with the concept of myself as "survivor". I hear how lucky I am, as I absorb horror stories and see why, at times, I have kept myself apart so as not to hear so much of what has happened to others, fearing it would lead me to think that the same could happen to me. I begin to feel there might be something in this to celebrate, that maybe I can receive what I have done. Might I pat myself on the back? I resonate to "The meek shall inherit the earth," and feel a cringe at the thought of 'standing out' in front.

I also learn that everyone attending the painting workshop but me had chemo every third week, instead of every other week. It may be easier and more sensible to do it that way, but it means six months of chemo, rather than four. I wanted to be finished by summer. Nine months of treatment is enough for me. I'm convinced I'll soon be firmly birthed into new health, with the umbilical cord of medical care cut and untied. Listening to the discussions, I'm also grateful I was able to have children, and that they are now grown. My path in this has been much easier than the path of others.

I also see that though I don't welcome death, I don't fear it in the way I used to. Even in my fatigue, I am aware that life balances on death, and I am currently centered in a series of enchanted rings.

April 24:

Today I'm full of life and love, even as fatigue is a mouse nibbling at my door.

April 25:

My breath moves in and out, a bird song on a day in spring. My radiation oncologist is thrilled with my progress. She says I'm the poster person for radiation energy. She's amazed. Though I figure she says that to everyone, I see myself on a poster bicycling with Lance Armstrong.

It seems that most people have trouble leaving radiation. There's an attachment to the attention. In the moment, I can't imagine it. I practically run out the door each day grateful to be free. I want to be ordinary and find delight in my ordinariness. I look between the leaves.

April 26:

I've been focused on being normal, and today someone asked what ordinariness means to me. This quote by Emily Dickinson comes to mind:

"To live is so startling it leaves little time for anything else."

I use stillness to renew. I feel the sky rest on the leaves of the tree, the trunk sink its roots into the ground.

April 27:

Someone brought donuts to radiation. It is a world of treats. Each day, I spend a little more time watching the fish. Also, today, though I usually look out on the garden from the waiting room, I turn and examine five watercolors on the wall. They are of five healing plants, and each one has dried plants from the Healing Garden I usually face. There is Taxol, Foxglove, Anemone Japonica, which is also known as Beauty Heals the Spirit, Echinecea, and Madagascar Periwinkle. When I compliment Francine on the care I'm receiving, she says the plants in the Wellness garden, and the whole building and everything in it, are gifts. As I leave, I read an Angel card from a bowl filled with stones. It was donated by a man in memory of his wife. It takes time to notice and absorb all the gifts that are here. Again, I see how it is up to me to be open and aware enough to receive.

The sun is out. What a difference the sun makes. I buy pink candles, purple iris, and a plant. I don't feel sick when I pass the meat in the grocery store. That's a step. I receive it like a kiss.

April 28:

When I come into the waiting room today, I look out at the Wellness garden and drink a mocha I make from the coffee and hot chocolate mix. Kirk feeds the fish. Steve, the nurse, passes through with warm robes. I noticed today there is a suggestion box and realized there is nothing I can suggest; I can only thank.

Despite that beginning, I'm tired by the time I get to the horses for my fourth session. Gisela suggests I visualize diving into and swimming in a pool of milk. She has been through many medical procedures and had three operations in one year, so she knows some tricks.

We work with the horses without a rope, using our body, gestures, and energy. We use the three steps: Ask, Suggest, Promise. I thought the third one was 'inspire', but it is promise. We promise that we mean what we ask.

I continue to be surprised at how well the horse obeys me when I know what I want. I don't speak; my presence is enough. I raise and lower my energy like a dimmer switch.

When I want the horse to come toward me, I step back, look at the horse's feet, and exhale. The horse, curious, comes forward to fill the space. If I stand there with my chest puffed out, where is the horse going to go? He'll head the other way. Jim talks about being on horse-time, which is slow to medium time. Most people today are on fast time, he says, and when nature is on fast time, it is a disaster. This is a time to slow, to fill. I am overflowing with love. Horse-time gives time to absorb.

April 30:

I pruned my plants today, really pruned. I used to trim gingerly. Now, I am Rambo. Whack! I am a person who has had her guts burned and returned. I understand root stock and strength. I know green sprouts within. I prune and trust what grows, revel in growth and return.

May 1:

I feel "normal" after my restful weekend, and so it feels odd to wake this morning and feel the lack of hair. I know I have said I have hair, and I do, but there is hair, a downy covering, and then there is something that flows; I am still waiting for a flow. There is nothing yet the wind can lift and swirl. In my dreams, I have hair.

It is beautiful outside, so I water the plants. Suddenly I notice that, in one day, hair has sprung forth on my arms and my legs. I am amazed. I wish the hair on my head would sprout as fast, but perhaps it is, and it is just less obvious up there, or maybe I expect more of the hair on my head.

Today a woman was playing the harp in the radiation waiting room. I sat there in my robe looking out at the garden. I was the only one there to listen and wrap in tears.

I am pretty blistered now, higher up than I expected to be. I haven't been rubbing the lanolin high enough. I didn't understand there are lymph nodes under the collar bone, and they are radiating me up to there. It will be a year before I can let the sun touch this whole area. I love the sun on my skin, so that is a long time to wait.

I'm realizing that I used to not know how I felt until I was over the top, either angry or sad, but I've become more sensitive. Today I feel sadness, just that, no story. I'm trying to take a longer view, to witness and to use my energy to do what I can do.

May 2:

My radiation appointment was long today, forty minutes with my arm over my head. I'm being prepared for my booster treatments, which will be more focused and intense. They wrote all over me, took pictures, and made a template. I have four more of the all over procedure, and then, drum roll, please, six boosters, which I'm hoping will be easier. The booster is focused in one spot, on the scar, rather than all over, which is now sore and blistered. I'm on schedule. My official ending celebration date is May 16.

I'm learning that the medical staff at the Marin Cancer Institute figured out how breathing protects the heart. They didn't get credit for this discovery, because they don't play 'the advertising game'. They don't even hand out free samples, because they don't believe in letting the pharmaceutical companies into the building. They aren't represented in *The New Medicine*, even though they are so terrific, because they don't hire publicists like some places do. So, this is my plug for Marin Cancer Institute, and the wonderful doctors and hearts that work there. I hope you don't need them, but if you do, they are there.

My hair is now long enough to swirl. It waves like dunes of sand.

My pruning has moved from gardens to closets and drawers. I have piles of stuff to give away. It feels symbolic of my hibernation and return. My color sense has changed. I'm attracted now to softer colors and peaches and pinks, like the gift of the sun as it rises and sets.

May 3:

I'm down to Number Ten in radiation treatments. A kindergarten teacher pointed out I have enough fingers to count down the remaining therapies. I'm holding all ten fingers up and tomorrow there will be nine. Hooray!

In cleaning out my closets, I decided that, from now on, I'm only going to wear what I really like. I used to save things for special occasions, but now every moment is special. I was a nature guide when my children were young. My teacher was Mrs. Terwilliger, who loved to run around the marsh, sand, and fields, shouting "Something special!" Life is like that, 'something special' all the time.

I woke this morning with Mandu resting on me, which is always a good excuse to stay in bed just a little bit longer. I thought about weight and gravity. When I studied Sensory Awareness with Charlotte Selver, we would pick up rocks and pass them to others, rocks of all shapes and sizes. This morning I begin to understand the importance of that, of using only the energy needed for each task, no more and no less. She would ask, "Are you all there for it?"

I think this experience has given me a better understanding of being all there for something, and also using the amount of energy needed, not too much and not too little, just right. Again, I am like Goldilocks, except without the curls, though they are on their way, I'm sure. I have enough eyelashes that I got to apply mascara this morning. This is exciting!

Then I went to radiation and again, set-up was pretty easy. They had country western music on today, and so I lay there, doing my breathing and listening to "She thinks my tractor is sexy." Well, we all learned something new. I relaxed so much listening to that song that they had to completely re-adjust me for the second part. My body just sank right down into the table. There has been a different CD on every time I go. Yesterday was Enya. My first time was Chopin, but today was the first time for country. I see now why parts of this country are sunk a bit low in the saddle. Listening to that music I let go. I could really feel it. Of course, a song about a tractor being sexy and the guy on it also being sexy...well, you too, would sink right into the table and let go. Whew!

I've never come out of the dressing room and stayed, but there is a young man who stays after his radiation treatment and works on the puzzle. Today the harpist was playing when I came out, and I told her what it meant to me to listen to her on Monday, and how sadness came up, just sadness, no story. She said that on Monday she was playing an old Hebrew song. Today she was just plucking what felt right to her. So this time, I stayed after treatment, and listened and talked to her. It seems they are starting a program to have people play the harp for those in the hospital. I suggested she play in the chemo room, and I told her about the view of Mount Tam.

Tonight I think about the words "sleep tight." I've always loved those words, but today, I'm thinking that perhaps it might be, "sleep loose." Isn't the open flower more able to beckon the bee and spread its pollen, like butter, on the bee's knees? I'm thinking I'll sleep loose tonight, spread out a bit, and lie on my back, visualize myself as a flower, welcoming the summer sun.

May 4:

I woke up in the night and went out to caress a new rose bush I purchased. I felt it needed comfort in its new home. It was shivering a bit in the wind and cold, though the sky was amazingly light in the night. I am peaceful and exuberant. I now have eight radiations left to go — two tough ones, and six easy ones. Hooray!

I feel like I'm standing on the edge of a pool, building up the courage to dive in. I shaved my legs for the first time in over five months. It was fun. I wore my wig to radiation and everyone loved it, though they also love my bare head. They think I should come wigless and hatless tomorrow. I'm hearing of more women who choose to have a double mastectomy and then reconstructive surgery, no radiation or chemo, rather than risk breast cancer. I wonder about it. I thought that possibility was not open to me, but I realize it may have been mentioned,

206

and I didn't take it in. I'm grateful to have my breasts, and I believe I chose the treatment that nourished me. Perhaps breasts are superfluous after a certain age, and yet, they don't feel so to me. I feel them as a warm couch.

We don't know what causes cancer, but the breast area seems especially vulnerable in this society. Yet, to remove them unnecessarily, to cook without the fire, I don't know. I have no answers. I just wonder how we balance what is lost, and I now know many women who do remove their breasts, and do it well with that, and even better than before. It is for each of us to choose.

I have not heard from Jane and it is okay. Our connection is irrelevant to time and space. I feel her as an opening. Her journey widens mine. We share the Japanese aesthetic of wabi-sabi, where beauty centers on impermanence and transience, and serenity is honored in change.

Looking Back: Cathy

My mind began to return with my hair, and I began to re-enter the world. I felt re-strung by the sound of the harp. I was interacting with others and learning more of journeys that paralleled mine. We each heard what we needed to hear to facilitate our own healing. I understood I had been living on 'horse time', and wondered how I could keep it integrated and viable in my newly expanding world.

Looking Back: Jane

When I returned from Spain, it took me a long time to call Cathy and check in. What I had experienced was beyond my expectations, and part of me was still under the spell. Of course, I also returned to find myself overtaken by my own life. There were piles of work to catch up on, hundreds of unread emails that demanded answering, and events in the life of my family that needed attention: a 'significant' birthday party to plan for my husband, my mother's preparations to make her last move, my son's decision about staying in school, and the news that my uncle had been diagnosed with cancer.

In truth, though, my biggest hurdle to calling wasn't any of these things. It was the feeling that for several weeks I had been able to experience my *own* life, fully and simply, without the overlay of another's real and daily need. I realized *I* had had enough. *I* was fatigued. *I* really didn't want to re-enter a world where cancer was the main character every day.

Those feelings were reinforced by another obstacle. Before leaving on my trip, I had been 'inside' Cathy's illness. I had been with her since the autumn and her discovery. Now I was outside. I no longer knew what Cathy needed. Things had happened I hadn't been part of. Others had probably stepped in. Not only that, but in a few short weeks, the perspective I'd gained while writing with Cathy - of seeing my own, everyday life as part of a continuum that included death — had faded. I had fallen into the myth that my life would go on forever in the rosy glow of being on vacation and traveling in a beautiful land.

Before I finally made the call to her, I spent some time reading her blog. I realized I was still a part of her story. I saw that Cathy had done well in my absence, and that she was in a different place now too. I knew there would be new aspects to our friendship and our writing partnership as well. I was able to call.

May 5:

I felt a bit odd today, as I now have only one more of the 'big guys.' I found myself lying there on the table awaiting radiation, remembering this journey that began last September. Soon I return to "normal." What does that mean? Was all of this normal? Can I stay present to my moods and needs? Will I know and say when I feel tired without the excuse of chemo and radiation?

All my friends in radiation world think I no longer need a hat, so I am considering unveiling at the stable today, though it is so cold right now, I may need a hat for warmth or sun. It is amazing what hair does. It is so useful, just like eyelashes and eyebrows. I am delighted to have hair, even though I thought I was doing just fine without it.

I open the windows so the plants can see in. I love how they peer in at me. They seem especially curious this morning. I gave them an extra dose of water. I believe they like me to water them personally rather than using the automatic sprinkler system. I understand. Imagine if the machine could set me up for radiation, instead of having two people checking and re-checking to make sure all is right. Twice, they put a rubber bib on me, and tuck it under my chin. It is very sweet. I am touched as they touch.

I return home between radiation and horses, so I'm less tired than I was last week. I want to be fresh for the horse experience, and I am. We practiced today with another human, as well as with the horses. When I was the horse, I felt the energy exchange, the unconscious response to the movement of the human. It was a lovely dance of give and take, ebb and flow. I am aware of fluidity in this world we share. There are no walls, no firm boundaries of where one begins and where another ends.

We humans sit in a circle at the start and conclusion of our experience with the horses. Emotions are close to the surface and much is shared. Jim, who leads the natural horsemanship group, says vulnerability is strength. We are vulnerable, and we are strong, both individually and as a group.

210

May 7:

I used to believe that life is based on a reward system. I figured if I was good enough', the cancer would be gone. I understand it isn't about that. I don't have control, but I have choice in my response. These words of Naomi Shihab Nye are my guide:

> *Walk around feeling like a leaf.*
> *Know you could tumble any second.*
> *Then decide what to do with your time.*

I check the moon tonight. The air is cool as I once again reflect on how the moon is always whole, though sometimes we see only a part. Sometimes I feel only one part of myself — only anger, or sadness, or fear, or joy — and yet, I am becoming more and more aware the whole is always there. Tomorrow is radiation. Only seven more to go!

May 8:

I go to radiation, my last 'Biggie', which is good, as I am experiencing some discomfort. "Lara's Theme" is the song for today. Tears come to my eyes as I lie there looking up at the lily pond that appears to float on the ceiling above. I see faces in the combination of water and water bugs. It's been a long time, and I'm weary and I appreciate how every effort is made to entertain us, to offer comfort and stimulation. Someone has thought of what the room is like from our point of view. I wonder if working with the horses has opened up my boundaries so I am more aware of what surrounds me, less caught up in all that has gone on within. Was I so aware of the contrasts and dimensions in the lily pond before? Did I see what was before me? Am I now able to open more places to explore? Can I take two dimensions and make them three, three and make them four? Are there more?

There was an elderly woman in the radiation room today. She had just had radiation, and was being taken upstairs for six hours of chemo. She was concerned about food. I told her husband he could bring food to her. Some do eat there, but I preferred to eat out afterward as my reward, and yet, she is having radiation and chemo at the same time and she is older than I. How will she do?

Seeing her, I was again aware how much we want to live. I would probably step right back into chemo if I had to, and yet, I wonder where it stops.

211

I rest this afternoon. I told my brother this has taken the wind out of my sails, and he said maybe it is time for me to drift, and so I do. I think I haven't really understood what happened, taken in that I've had cancer. Perhaps the time is coming to get in touch with all I have been through.

May 9:

In the moment, all is well, though somehow the set-up for the next stage was not right, so after much probing, marking, checking, re-checking, and consulting, everything needed to be done again, which meant I didn't have radiation today. Now I'll end next Wednesday, May 17, not Tuesday, the 16th. It is fine, yet today was not so pleasant. I'm very sore. I went without a hat, and everyone loved it, so no more hats except for when I'm in the sun, or when I'm cold. What a relief! Step by step, I return to life as it was before.

May 10:

I am thrilled that Jane and I again commit to our morning writing. I could have written while she was gone, but didn't, and so it is. We support each other in writing our morning flow.

I'm feeling a bit demoralized, and am in physical discomfort. They put a metal strip over the scar before they take a picture. Having that taken on and off yesterday, and all the marking and pushing on an already-sore area, has me feeling a wee bit miserable this morning. I have to laugh as I read my friend Vicki's comments on how up-beat I've been. I feel myself losing it a bit today. I'm hoping for an easy day.

Today was painful like yesterday. I felt like I was in a torture chamber. I wish I was better prepared for this part. I realize each person's response to radiation and pain is different, but I think hearing that this was supposed to be the easy part didn't prepare me for what was to come. The problem is that any touch is painful right now, even my soft camisole. Therefore, the need to place a piece of metal over the scar and poke and write on me, and then put plastic on me and write some more, is hard, but the template is now done. It is a piece of lead shaped just for me so I am radiated in just the right place. Francine doesn't work on Tuesdays, so I was a little worried that a doctor I didn't know decided the new template was okay, but then I realized how much they all care. I continue to be held in fine hands.

212

I learned today that the computers are so exact, that the treatments are never exactly the same amount of time. Although the power or force is programmed in, the treatment is affected by the temperature and humidity of the room, and so it takes everything into account and gives just the "right" amount.

I appreciate all these people running around and checking that everything is just right, and treating me like a celebrity, yet even so, today, I felt like crying. I was literally shaking while trying to stay still. The radiation is cumulative even after it is done, so it's continuing to worsen and will continue to do so, even though certain parts of me are not being radiated now. I realized when I looked in the mirror that I am burned. When Mary Pat, the nurse, checked me today, she gave me a new ointment to use instead of the Lanolin. It's Aquaphor, and I'll use it over the hydrocortisone for the next two-and-a-half to three weeks. The problem is mostly where I have been sunburned in the past. That area raises and new skin forms underneath, so when this heals, I'll peel and have a new layer of skin in some places. There are women who have been sunburned over the whole breast. Try to imagine that. I feel like an ad for covering up. It is easy to stay away from the touch of the sun right now.

I had radiation today, too, which also was painful. It took a minute after a set-up of probably thirty minutes. But the good news was that Dan had an opening for a massage today. I hadn't returned to him because I thought I was doing so well, and I didn't want to take the time. But today and yesterday I haven't been doing so well, so I appreciate the opening.

I've been reading a book on communicating with dogs, so I nodded a "hello" to Ralston, Dan's seeing-eye dog, as I came in. He rose and came right over and gave me a full-on kiss, something that dogs, I now know from the book, *The Other End of the Leash*, rarely do. They usually approach from the side. While Dan was out of the room, I told Ralston how pitiful I felt.

Then I told Dan that I was feeling miserable. I felt guilty last time complaining, because Dan is legally blind. Today, I felt lousy enough to confide how badly I felt. I see the burns. It was painful to lie on my stomach, but we made it work. It's an upper body massage, and I felt how tense I've been. I let go. He held my head. I felt like a cave with new openings. Pain does route out new space for joy.

Dan said he learned a new quote. It was something about cremating disappointment, rather than embalming it. It was appropriate, as I've been feeling disappointed that my 'ending' is not quite as I had

213

envisioned. I wanted to float out of radiation on wings. I felt today like I was crawling out on my knees. These last few days have been important. I'm feeling what I have been through, how long it has been, and how much I want it to be done.

Here are our poems from this morning, Jane and mine. We're back in our flow. Poetry is a lovely way to speak, comfort and entice release.

Conducting

> *so many kinds of pain,*
>
> *in one body -*
>
> *a symphony today -*
>
> *the rash has its own tone,*
>
> *a grating sound,*
>
> *like a stick drawn across a board*
>
> *shaped like a porcupine,*
>
> *each quill sharp and fast as a 32nd note.*
>
> *The swelling is a drum.*
>
> > *Boom, Boom, Boom.*
>
> *The scar is a triangle.*
>
> > *Ting, Ting, Ting.*
>
> *The underarm is a violin,*
>
> > *long notes lifted like lace to the sky.*
>
> > *Gut no longer believes in a grand finale.*
>
> > *Cello come in,*
>
> > > *as tears fall,*
>
> *pluck, pluck, pluck, the strings of a harp.*

— Cathy

214

It would be like daylight savings time, twice a year.

We'd pick a moment, maybe the first second of each solstice
When midnight arrives in a boat on the New Zealand coast.
Wherever we'd be - each of us - we'd sit.
On the first out breath we'd all say ONE.
We'd do this - all of us - for twenty minutes.
For awhile we'd all be in rhythm like seaweed in the current
Sighing together until the next time.

— Jane

May 11:

I am in some discomfort this morning, and I feel how the pain keeps me present. I am right here, in this moment, nowhere else. Perhaps that's a good thing. It's like a little hammer thumping, "Now, Now, Now."

So at radiation, I point out that I am in pain, and I say I'm trying to understand why these last treatments were supposed to be easier. I say those words as the machine is rammed in tightly against me, and my arm is pulled up even more to make room for it. Ah, I misunderstood. Not easier, so it seems, but different! Now I don't have to control my breathing, and once the machine is set up, there is a one- minute blast at a focused area, and that is it. The machine isn't moved around me, and I'm not radiated from different places. Now I understand that different is *not* easier. In addition to the one-minute blast, there is still the writing on me, which is very painful at this point, as well as the manipulation; and yes, I will continue to get sorer. The effects are cumulative, and the discomfort continues after I think I'm done. It is like the eyelashes falling out after my last chemo. I will get more and more 'radiant'. I am happy to know I glow the dark.

This procedure takes less time though, so I hit traffic both ways. Today, when I'm finished, I get in the car with a brownie in my hand, since it's another woman's last day of radiation, and she brought treats. It seems many of us are finishing near the same time, but there will be a new crop to replace us. On the car radio, a man is giving his comment on his chemo experience. He has a lot of 'D' words to describe it. I can only remember some of them: dismal, depressing, debilitating, and

215

disastrous. He speaks of feeling left out, and wondering if he is doing the right thing. He says if he weren't doing chemo, he would feel good. He could be in Hawaii drinking Mai Tai's. "Why am I doing it?" he asks, and then he says he has always been a gambler, but he never expected to be playing Russian roulette. My feelings exactly! I drive out of the Marin Cancer Institute, over the speed bump, and make my right turn listening to his chemo complaints. No wonder I feel so sad, brutalized, and traumatized. I was too sick to feel this way before, but I feel well enough to feel it now.

My hair is coming in, and people are complimentary, but I don't look like the person I remember. One woman told me not having hair saves her twenty minutes a day. I look at myself, and say yes, it's an interesting look, this new, short hair, but I realize I never had time to grieve the loss of my hair, to say "good-bye" to that happy, carefree woman who's no longer here. It isn't that I'm not happy, and of course, I say I am joyous, as joy contains the sorrow, but there is a new gravity. The lightness has more depth, more shadow, and I have more wrinkles. I decide to view wrinkles as trees, knowing the light needs trees to hold and display it, to lift it like a ballerina, so shadows can play with leaves.

And still I grieve. Though we tried to create some rituals to say goodbye to my hair, I see now it was false in its gaiety. We shared a vessel of shock.

I ground now, ground my sorrow, grieve the woman I was, or at least the woman I remember I might have been. I remember there was a time during treatment when I had no tears. I felt chemo dried them up. But radiation is letting them flow. Four more treatments to go, a couple more weeks of pain, I'm told, and in a month, I "should" feel pretty good. I'm sure that will be so.

I saw Dr. Susan Myers today, an acupuncturist and Naturopathic doctor. My purpose in seeing her was to deal with the numbness and tingling in my feet, but I see that it's time to more fully step into another kind of doctoring. She confirmed how traumatic radiation is, saying I was cut, poisoned, and burned. She is clear: "cut, poisoned, and burned". Through her, I feel what I've been through. Later I learn she knows what she is talking about. She has been through it, too.

Lying on the table, the first thing I noticed was that I could lie there and turn my head to the right, as a baby would do when it feeds. It felt so important to be able to turn my head after twenty-nine treatments of radiation, where my head lay, held in a little metal basket, looking

216

straight up, not supposed to move. We endure a great deal to ensure that we live.

I also learned today how out of touch with my own breath I have become, with so many orders on how to breathe in order to move my heart out of the way to accommodate the machine. That's a nerve-wracking experience, especially for someone who wants to do everything just right, like I do. The acupuncture helped me release. I lay on the table with my teeth chattering, tears falling first from the right eye and then the left. It is as though, piece by piece, I was being unfrozen from the rigidity that has carried me through.

I've also been surprised to see how much harder it is to think healing thoughts when the radiation blaster is continuously right up against my skin. Before, it was only on me for around 36 seconds, then about ten, and then it proceeded to move back and forth between ten and 36-second intervals. It may sound odd, but a minute, under such circumstances, is a long, long time. I feel myself tensing to get away from the blast from the machine. Again, this is not such a healthy thing.

Dr. Myers emphasized how my cells are being destroyed, and how I need more rest to heal, so I have a prescription for naps. I walked out of her office carrying a flotilla of vitamins, minerals, and herbs.

I'm starting to feel what I've been through, this medical treatment of surgery, chemo, and radiation. I've been a good soldier throughout. That was necessary, but now, I feel that I can begin to let go. I also plan to create a more welcoming image for the machine as I further integrate the concept of self-care.

A woman who worked with me today was upset that her cousin chose chemo over a trip to Italy with his family, when he was told he only had a few more months to live. I tried to explain to her how strong the desire to live is. I've been stunned at what I've accepted in my desire to live. Once, when I was in the Everest region of Nepal, I crawled — literally crawled — to the altitude sickness clinic. I do it again.

May 12:

I'm feeling well this morning, and I've worked with my attitude so I can again view radiation as healing energy coming my way. I think the difficulties this week with the template, which led to more manipulation than usual, were upsetting. Also, everything is discussed in front of me. I need to be there, so I hear, "Do you think it is right?" and, "Are you sure it is right?" It is reassuring that the medical staff is so careful, yet equally

217

disconcerting to know that it is not an exact science, and is subject to human error. There is no 'perfect' here, nor is there anywhere, but sometimes it is comforting to think that there is, and again, the intensity of care is overwhelmingly cautious and dear.

As Jane and I spoke this morning, I remembered the other day, when two policemen led a prisoner out of the cancer center. He was shackled and looked embarrassed in his orange suit, walking between the two men in uniform. I felt sorry for him. He seemed so naked in the bright light.

In the acupuncture session when I released energy I had been holding, I felt how I had built a container for myself, a prison. I set myself in a stoic, rigid position to carry myself through the medical procedures. My jaw was tight and my head held high. I did not allow myself to cry at the treatment center. What did that take? I was finding out now. I wonder how our prison system would be if we offered acupuncture as a way for prisoners and guards to release their energy, anger, frustration, sorrow, fear, and pain. Perhaps we could let them work with horses and dogs. What if this that I am receiving was offered to others in a different kind of need? What if prisoners and guards had a stronger system of support?

Today I am told that I am a difficult case. Because of the shape of my scar, the severity of my problem, and the odd angles, a doctor came over from the hospital to ensure all was okay. Three doctors have checked me this week. The doctor touched me gently as he introduced himself, and the others touched me as we waited for him to come. I felt treasured, and because of that, there was no pain. I see how psychological pain can be. I was ready for the radiation treatment today, prepared, and it went both easily and well. I picked up a stone from the altar at the entry. I have it here with me. Today was Number Thirty. I am grateful there are only three more sessions to go.

Today has been incredibly affirming, and again, I went without a hat, and everyone loves my hair and my new 'look'. It seems I am "chic and hip". I read the latest news on breast cancer treatment, which is changing so that for women like me, chemo may not be necessary in the next few years. I am grateful for that.

It is my sixth time with the horses, and we are riding now. When I first got on top of the horse, I was holding the horn of the saddle with my right hand, while my left hand was clenched. Kim pointed out my clenched left hand, and when I released it, my whole upper body relaxed. I sway now, even in my chair, mobile and relaxed, living as massage. It is an important lesson in noticing what I'm doing with my hands, whether on a horse or not.

Radiation - The Boosts

The radiation machine is pushed against my side,
my arm pulled up over my head.
I struggle to visualize this intense penetration,
which I am told is actually more shallow,
as healing energy.
I am sore.
I see what radiation can do.
This is not a play.
Jane suggests Tai Chi, changing the energy.
I lean into that, counter attack
with a move of my own.
I block, shift, turn, change, hop, direct,
like with the horses
when we place our body so they go around,
or with dogs where we deflect
their exuberance
with hips and shoulders.
I work today with the energy from the machine like that.
I have tools.
I am biological. Adapt!

— Cathy

I read the news: Moussaoui moves to Supermax.

The shoe bomber, the UNAbomber, the Oklahoma bomber
They all are there.
They say it is worse than dying:
Eighty-four square feet, no sky and no connection,
No way to catch the tears, channel the chatter, transform the nerve.
Each one melts into a pool of their own wax.
Permanently alone.

- Jane

Looking Back: Cathy

We work so hard to save a life like mine, and yet, we judge and kill. Is one life worth more than another? How do I pay back this gift? I wish everyone in the world could have this much care. Imagine if each child were so gently touched and told daily by so many your life matters this much.

Community carried me through. From earliest times, shunning has been a punishment. Banned from the tribe a person cannot survive.

Looking Back: Jane

On my return, I realized how outward my view had become. While I'd been sightseeing, Cathy had continued to listen, adjust, master the machine, and track an invasion of her body that she hadn't asked for. She was allowing what her body needed.

I had been away from that shared cocoon, was out in the world listening to the news, much more than I had been before my trip. I was beginning to sense that my writing was taking me new places. I wondered if my current perspective would create a distance between us. Could I be with Cathy again in a way that was supportive, while still being true to where my attentions were taking me?

Mother's Day

May 13:

I go outside to honor my mother, doing so by placing two pink roses and a new stone in the bird bath I purchased in her memory. I wrap pink jasmine around the base, and plant purple pansies. I miss my mother this Mother's Day weekend. Last year I was still actively grieving, and this year, I feel her spirit, her tender, joyful being, and how very much I miss her.

Though we don't wear black in this country as was done in the past, I think a black armband could announce to others that we are grieving and need special care.

May 14:

I remember Mother's Day when Jeff and Chris were young. I would hear them in the kitchen with Steve, making breakfast for me to eat in bed. One would go out and pick a flower for the vase. Then, they would watch me eat. I would feel so guilty, and then, there would be a whole day that was mine. Whatever I wanted, they would provide. They were so enthusiastic in their giving, in their joy. I had trouble receiving that. I kept thinking I should carry something, or wash a dish. I wouldn't have trouble with that today. I've learned to receive, and in that, I can take care of myself, better care than before. This morning I woke, and then went back to sleep, and then woke again and did the same. It was delicious. When I woke the last time, I realized that each one of us tends to mother others when we take care of our families and friends. I'm speaking of both males and females here. Let's all today take some moments to mother ourselves. Every day is Mother's Day for me now. I am well-cared for today and every day. Those who get breast cancer are often care-givers. Let's each learn to receive.

May 15:

Two more radiations to go. Hooray! When I took my shower this morning, there was pain when water hit my underarm on the left side. When I asked about it, they told me it will get worse.

My brother writes to say he and my niece Katy attended the Yankees game in New York on Saturday. For Mother's Day and breast cancer awareness, the players wore pink wrist bands, pink ribbons, and some of the players used pink bats!

It has been almost eight months of medical care. I have been trying not to get too excited, but when I'm asked how it feels to have only two more days, I feel the prison gate open to a magic garden, where I step in carefully. I am a ballerina with long, delicate toes, feeling my way.

The end of treatment is like:

walking on a trampoline.

living at the North Pole with Santa, reindeer, and elves.

feeling the ice caps firm enough for polar bears to feed, breed, and roam.

flying a hang-glider and landing easily to stand, wings spread like a bird.

running on sand, bouncing in waves, and swimming upstream to breed.

Awe

> *the starting point of consciousness*
> *where the breath comes in*
> *and touches the heart of our lungs*
> *like the hummingbird beak*
> *the place where pistil and stamen meet.*
>
> *The ovary is a bulb.*
>
> *Squeeze and release*

— Cathy

My mother taught me to fold men's shirts in half lengthwise down the middle, matching shoulder seams and sleeves, then doubling the shirt twice more into a tidy rectangle. But the last time, folding my father's just-dried shirts, unsure why we had washed them in the first place, I folded them in half widthwise, the sleeves crucified, so I could press my palms across his chest again.

— Jane

Looking Back: Cathy

I was ecstatic with anticipation for the end of radiation. I couldn't know that I would soon feel I had been dumped off the track I had been pulled along for so long, and left to sit in neutral trying to remember how to put myself into gear.

Looking Back: Jane

All bodies are new every seven years, we're told. No cell of mine is the same today as it was seven years ago. Could I observe these minute changes if I paid closer attention, as Cathy did through her treatment?

And what of stories and memories? Do these die with the cells that held them? Did treatment change Cathy's memories? Are we human because of our stories? Would we still be human without our stories? Are stories like bridges to carry us across the unknown in our lives? Could letting go of our stories, as our bodies let go of the memories of pain, make us more human?

There is no end, only beginning.

May 16:

In the night, I was so excited that I had trouble sleeping. I have only two radiations left, one today at 8:30, and one tomorrow at noon.

Anna from radiation said I'm a good sport. I'm good at staying still. The machine and I are the best of friends. Anna worried about the machine pinching my arm, but nothing could affect my day. I was floating on clouds.

It was my checkout day from radiation, even though I have one more procedure. I met with Dr. Poen, who is gentle, tender, and radiates joy. When I told him that, he said these attributes are present in all the people in that department, and he is right. It is a radiant place, in all ways. Mary Pat gave me my final instructions. I am welcome to return if I need help. I breathe that in, happy today.

Afterwards, I met my friend Penny, who is visiting from New York. Together we celebrated my first trip to the beach at Tennessee Valley, me in two sun-proof hats and a sun-proof jacket. My heart exulted to be in my favorite place, with all the greens and beginnings of gold. We met a fine quail. I walked right into the ocean and baptized myself. My head is refreshed. Walking back, we saw what could only be a river otter in the lagoon. It was unbelievable. What a day!

Stanley Kunitz, a wise man and poet who died two days ago on May 14, after living to be one hundred, wrote that, "The deepest thing I know is that I am living and dying at once, and my conviction is to report that dialogue."

For a moment, the sky opens, and I see the moon. It's like that, isn't it, light and dark, life and death? I accept that I'm "living and dying at once", and in this moment, I'm lifted in the holy arms of life, like a baby, and kissed. The moon plays games, peek-a-boo and hide-and-seek. I am a cauldron in which life and death simmer and brew and I'm held in a wider cauldron too.

May 17:

When I woke, I felt like a little kid on her first day of school. I was up early, goodies bought and ready to share. Yesterday Dr. Poen, (I always want to type 'Poem') spoke of what a privilege it is to work with people who have been through chemo and are now going through radiation. I think I got what a 'special' group I've been in, and will always be in. Most of us, I believe, were raised to fear cancer, but now it provides a chance to live the juxtaposition of being inward and outward, with time and support to cocoon, rest, reflect. As he talked, I felt that even if I had died, this would have been worth it. But Dr. Poen assured me I'm here to live a long, long time.

Jane asks what this means. It means that treatment is done. I assure her I am fine. Mandu has his head on my hand. He likes to warm my hand as I type. He's suggesting there might be better things to do than type, like pet him. He's purring, though, so I guess all is okay.

I dress carefully for today, as though I were a priest or priestess of long ago. I comb my hair. The ritual is important. Grooming ourselves means we are well, and I am well. I am well, healed, whole!!

I stop at the bakery for cookies. Before, I would have baked them. Now, I buy them, honoring self-care and recognizing that the gift, the offering, the intention are born and nurtured inside.

Since my appointment time is later today, I have time to prepare for my last treatment, my stepping out of one world and into another. I remember a dream of years ago, where I lifted up a man-hole cover, and peered out on a wide, flat plain. Perhaps this is that as I step up and out.

This last treatment is a holy rite. Perhaps they all were, and now I know. I create an altar in the waiting room and light votive candles that I place in candle holders of yellow, blue, green, and red. I place a giggling, sparkly stuffed bee on the altar, and two decks of cards, one of "52 Things to Try Once in Your Life," and the other "52 Ways to Celebrate Friendship." Hasn't that been what this journey has been? Each day has been something new I've tried, and this is a true celebration of friendship at the deepest levels. I spread out chocolate letters spelling out "Thank You", and chocolate hearts, wrapped in red and gold.

The nurse, Steve, looks at all I've done and speaks to me in a way I haven't heard from him before. He says he prays each day for all of us that come here, that he views this as a healing place, a temple, mosque, or church.

My giggling bee was a hit, and is now on the mirror, so when people walk into the radiation room, they can squeeze his tummy and hear him giggle.

There was one amazing hitch. I went in and lay down perfectly. I have it figured out for the thirty-third time, so there is no need to adjust; they mark away, set it all up, and leave the room. There is a little click-y sound as it programs, and then, everything dies, except the lights, which come on because they're on a generator. Unbelievable! So as I lie there with my arm up, they go to get the physicist, who fixes it, and away we go. But for more than a moment, I thought tomorrow was going to be the last day, rather than today. I could only laugh. It seemed so funny, and that is what I am noticing. I like to laugh. I remember being outside the monastery at Tengboche at 13,000 feet in Nepal, hearing all this laughter from the monks as they sat inside and ate. I thought they would be sober and quiet, but they appear to worship on the belly laugh. I like it, and this lack of exercise has given me quite a soft belly with which to jiggle and laugh. I am JOY!!

Also, I rolled my eyes back when I was lying on the table, and what did I see? There is a dragonfly up there, on the ceiling, in the marsh, a copper one, attached by a magnet to the metal that defines the ceiling. Amazing!! I had not noticed the dragonfly before today. Maybe it's taken this long to believe I've been given back my wings.

I walk out, an inspiration for those sitting there in turbans and hats. I'm done.

Leaving, I noticed Kirk, one of the technicians, owner of the parrot and feeder of the fish. He was playing Solitaire on the computer. What a combination of modern technology and actual physical touch this experience has been. I am a product of the best of both worlds, natural and man-made.

I meet Chris for lunch at Noonan's in Larkspur Landing. We share some tears, bittersweet. I have two glasses of French champagne. When else am I ever going to have so much to celebrate? I'm satiated and I have time for all that I could ever want. I come home and read the notes on my graduation certificate, again, deeply touched.

The Dalai Lama says, "It's best not to get too excited or too depressed by the ups and downs of life." I agree. I am calm. When the computer went down for the radiation machine today, I stayed calm, knowing I could come back the next day, and the day after that. What I am doing in each moment is just right for me. Just the gift of life is enough.

229

The Day of my last Cancer Treatment

Today I stand in a field like a horse.

There are no fences.

*I gallop, canter, and trot, knowing I am a herd
      animal.*

I ground and fill my spot.

With wolves, the omega is grieved the most.

The whole tribe gathers, sorrows for the loss.

*The alpha only leads, but the tail tells where we've
      been,*

is scribe for the heart.

— Cathy

230

Looking Back: Cathy

There is no end. What is head or tails for the coin that is tossed? Each landing brings something new to view. I stretch on stars, climb a jungle gym of light.

Looking Back: Jane

Seven months together almost every morning, and now, here is the end.

While I don't think this is the end of either Cathy's or my stories, it does feel like a new beginning. Now is the time for each of us to be with this new manifestation of our friendship, to see how we have been changed by the unexpected gifts that cancer has brought.

The End/No End

May 18:

I woke this morning remembering the children's story *Good Night Moon*. I felt like I was in my own story — *Good Morning Room*. I opened my eyes and looked at everything around me individually, and said, "Good Morning." I slept long and deeply, and I have no pain this morning. The day is before me.

I am learning to just be. Today Karen said it might be time for some fun, and I found myself struggling with the word 'fun'. What does that mean? I'm not quite sure anymore, and maybe that is the place where fun comes and taps me on the shoulder, and is delighted to find me. Can I open to receive this thing called 'fun'?

May 19:

It has been quite the day. I rose and quickly posted on my blog, did the free flow writing with Jane, scurried to Muir Beach for a shower at Karen's, since the gas connection to my house suddenly went out and I have no heat or hot water, and there I enjoyed seeing Karen, a view, having a hot shower and then some tea. After breakfast with Jeff at the Rain Tree Cafe, I drove up to Fairfax to see the horses. We sat in a circle under the trees, and one woman shared that she walks through Whole Foods with a hat on her head, wearing it like a set of blinders to dampen some of the stimulation of the store. I don't think we realize how bombarded we are until we go through something like this.

Today was another glorious horse day. Last week at the stables, Kimberly had taken photos of me hugging the horse, Flamin', and she gave them to me today. I realize it is my first time seeing myself in a photo with a little bit of hair. I look happy.

Today we learned to guide the horse with our 'sit bones'— that bony part of ourselves we often ignore as we slump instead of sitting firmly upright. When we are in contact with the horse with our sit bones and sink down, the horse stops, and we rest as one. It is as easy at that.

Hallie, my horse for today, knew I wanted to kiss her, and she kept coming forward for a kiss. She was happy to oblige. It is about my intention. The horse does what I desire her to do. Unfortunately, I seem unable to mobilize much desire for the horse to do anything but snuggle. I'm supposed to be decisive and direct left or right. We practice feeling the place of neutrality, so we can raise and lower our energy when needed. I am again reminded of my work with Charlotte Selver, where we practiced learning to use the energy needed for the task at hand — no more and no less. The horses know when we are in our heads and not our bodies, when we leave the place of unknowing and try. It is instant feedback. As somatic workers know, "The body doesn't lie." The horses want us to lead from that confident place of the body, not that illusive, trickster place of the mind. We have to come into our bodies to work with the horses, and it is obvious to ourselves and others when we do, and when we don't. There is no place to hide here.

At first, it was painful for me to pull my left arm out to lead the horse, but now I move my arm easily. My sternum is forward and out, responding to the love that is here. I give thanks for all who have come together to create and give the gift of equine therapy to my friends and me.

Again, One

People who only know me with no hair,
and hats, think I look beautiful,
but my friends who knew me before
still look shocked - who am I, so soft, tender, and scared -
tears come like opossums in the night -
marsupial am I - my pouch holds shards of fear.
I wash them in the stream, and all disappears

— Cathy

233

Looking Back: Cathy

I had been a person in treatment. Who was I now? It was curious that the gas connection to the house wore out at this time, and needed a new valve. What was that saying to me?

I remember reading that the cervix needs several years to stabilize after having a pap test. At times, I still shake and shiver as though I am on the table with a huge machine wrapped around me.

I found myself, at this time, seeking the domesticity of the plants in my yard. I would open the windows and invite the plants to peer in. I go to them when I'm upset.

My dreams were telling me I was enough. In my dreams, I didn't need a house, and yet, when awake, I did. I had to fix what had broken. The world of spirit could no longer carry me. It was time for my feet to touch and stroke the ground. It was also time to recognize the valve was replaced and turn on the gas.

Looking Back: Jane

The horse experience had happened mostly without me because I was traveling when it began. When Cathy reexamined the horse experience and realized what it had held for her, I understood a little more about my presence and my role as a support during Cathy's illness.

I realized that, in some ways, I had been like the horse. I had responded to Cathy's physical moods and sensations; I had been there, listened to her, and watched. Even my writing had changed in response to her. The material that came to me was less about my own path or journey, as much of my poetry in the past had been. Instead, it had taken on the form that emerged in January during Cathy's illness. In retrospect, these poems for me feel like responses to the situation of Cathy's illness, in much the same way the horse responds to the presence of a human — instinctive, watchful, cautious, while at the same time, seeking to establish trust.

It has taken a little longer for me to understand how the year I spent writing with Cathy has changed me. But from the vantage point of time, there are at least two things that seem significant. Before Cathy's illness, I had never made time for my writing, even though writing has been a part of my life since I was small. Now, although we still honor it, the writing I do with Cathy in the morning is not the only time I write. I give whole weekends to myself, and will often carve out an evening or two every week to writing. But perhaps even more significant to me, I have seen and felt how being– just *being* and not doing, just paying attention, even without writing– is a way to be in this world. I experience this way of being as having a wholeness with myself and with my life that was not there before. That is the piece of this experience I treasure most.

May 20:

The equine therapy program, like many programs these days, needs to raise money, so I volunteer to help staff a booth at a summer fair in Fairfax on June 11. I want to give something back. I feel rested this morning, truly rested, and sort of plumped up, like a pillow. My cells are awake and full, not drooping like wilted flowers.

I feel my feet on the floor today. They still feel gritty, like I'm walking on sand. I hope that will go away. I'm amazed how long I am affected by Taxol. But I'm sleeping more and deeper, while also feeling the increasing light of these late May days fertilize my bones.

May 21:

Treatment doesn't stop with the end. It's like halting a huge barge. The effects are cumulative. My feet still tingle, and yet, at the stables, I am able each time to open out my left arm even wider. I can lead the horse without pain. My hair returns more and more each day, and energy comes in to dance and play.

May 24:

I had an acupuncture session today to try and deal with this issue with my feet. I'm doing much better since last time I went, though my lung meridians are down. The lungs hold grief. She said I feel traumatized because I am choosing to let go, and by letting go, I feel more. Some choose never to feel what happened, but since I choose to do so, I need to be kind to myself. She reminded me of my prescription for naps. I forgot after two days of them, and am now tired.

Tonight I feel like a newly-born foal, ready to stand and nuzzle. New places are being born in me, new stars.

For Jim McDermott, Mentors, and Horses of Marin Stables

I struggle to write what you mean to me,

to put my right brain in the reins of the left

and say this is about balance and neutrality,

raising our energy and lowering it,

responding to demand and need.

This is about trust.

I lost so much this year, every hair.

I felt bare, naked. My eyes seemed huge,

and hugeness is still there, in horse eyes, horse heart.

I feel secure as though I have four legs,

and when I ride on the back of a horse,

supported by horse lungs and sit bones

I feel aligned. Horse time.

— Cathy

May 26:

Today was another magical day with the horses, a day of receiving even more gifts. Before we close our circle for the final time, I ride like the wind and post easily. I am on Hallie again. We are friends. I think it should be called 'Hug Therapy', since there are so many. We are a circle of love. I have learned to use my energy in a soft, yet assertive way, to direct and guide, and to know what I want, so I can get it. I am grateful for all the work that brought these volunteers together at Marin Stables in Fairfax, for Jim McDermott, Cindi Cantrill, Diane Brandon, and all the others, both human and horse.

May 30:

Jane and I talk this morning about "being special." When I was in the medical world, I was 'special.' Now, I am just one of many, and that is special, too. Here is Jane's beautiful, sweet poem on being special, and yes, her name is Hope.

Hope is the flower girl.

She has a yellow dress, orange socks, and red hair.
She is softly singing about rainbows and sunshine.
Her tiny arms are curved in balletic arcs.
Her toes inside her rounded canvas shoes are pointed, just so.
She wishes the bride whose shower this is
A happy wedding marriage.
Then she curtsies,
Pulls up her dress, adjusts her panties.

— Jane

Life -

the shine of newly written ink on a page in the sun

moments of liquid, caught

before they're gone

— Cathy

June 8:

I take an online test about personal boundaries, and see that I am more connected than I was before, and my boundaries are stronger. I now know in and out, what is mine, and what I share with others. I have more awareness of choice.

Jane and I reflect back, and realize we began with me as the still point around which Jane revolved. We each, at times, envied the other. Now we each can be still, and we both revolve and interact in the world.

Now not only is my hair long enough to comb, but it is long enough to have a direction. I think the reason people noticed my eyes so much when I had no hair was because there was no distraction of direction. The point was clear. Here are two eyes. "Enter here."

I now know that many people start blogs as a way to deal with their illness. Jane and I look back and see that this is a journal of presence. We are grateful for the opportunity to journey and journal both together and apart.

Life goes on:

My dear friend Cat Mandu died easily June 22. I felt he absorbed the poisons of my treatment and helped carry me through. I didn't think I could have another pet after such a huge loss, but, on August 8, I woke and felt drawn to go to the Humane Society. There were Tiger and Bella, siblings in a cage, with Tiger at the front like a carnival hawker, and Bella hunkered frightened and small in the back. I brought them home, and Bella went right to Mandu's spot on the bed. Mandu's body is buried in the yard, and his spirit romps here as our guide and friend.

Jeff and Jan were married September 10. Soon after, I participated in a fashion show for breast cancer survivors. We were all beautiful. Many were shockingly young. It was a huge bonding and success. We danced well into the night. It signaled an end.

One time, I walked down Mt. Tamalpais from Pantoll, past the tree that was one of my guides, to Stinson beach. I walked right into the ocean in my clothes. When I emerged, a young boy came up to me with a towel. That is how generously life provides. I again carry a purse. Jane's comb from Spain resides inside. I continue to strive to fulfill the words of the Dalai Lama: "My religion is very simple. My religion is kindness."

When I began to feel truly healed, Jane and I drove up the mountain and walked on the slopes that slant west. We then went up to the top and circled around. We climbed up to the tip-top where the fire look-out sits. All fires were out and the view was clear.

The End of Beginning

Sometimes a door shuts, so softly the air barely whispers

It seems a small thing, the pull of hydrogen, carbon

Then you notice that something you've known all your life has gone missing.

Like an ear that goes deaf, a dog that's gone lost— here and then not.

It seems a large thing, the attraction of carbon to carbon.

You spend some time feeling the edges this something fits into,

Something whose secrets you've held in your throat, here and then not,

Know the shape of your loss against sky til its absence is no longer new.

You spend some time missing the spaces that held it.

Still alive in your cells, in the bright flash of memory

You sing for the missing until being gone is something forgotten

Except for the lightning it makes through your limitless dreams.

Still alive in your cells, in the you that is past

The scent you've rubbed in your palms now is absent

Except in the tangle of vast inner space.

Sometimes a door opens on a landscape unknown.

Oxygen cracks with the scent of ozone and salt.
Now the ground softens, the air opens outward
You pass through the door, embracing the space
Where gravity loosens its grip on your footsteps.

Now the hills melt, the air becomes rare
Your lungs are balloons from which you're suspended
And gravity loses its grip on your feet.
There is nothing around to signify human.

Your lungs become wings with which you can fly
Below there's no tree, no house and no person
There is nothing around not even a stranger
By which to measure your rise and your fall.

Below and above is a landscape of light
No hunger or loss or understood language
By which to measure your joy or your fear.

It's a small thing. It's simple. You're free.

- Jane

When the Rules Seem to Change

When the lantern on the hill

to which you looked to climb

is extinguished,

you are back to candlelight.

Pour wax over a wick, and strike,

know light from the inside out,

the glow so bright it seems like night,

and the stars spin within.

- Cathy

Lagunitas Creek

I enter a living redwood tree,

opened to an inner pyramid by fire,

sit on a root with Jane.

We share a stage coach,

watch the passing landscape,

from the vantage point of a tree.

The oceans hold streams

like jump ropes.

The song is begun.

Harmonize with the leaves.

- Cathy

Background:

I met Jane in a workshop called Eyes of the Beholder. It was created by Karen Roeper and Jane as a way to see one's 'self' more kindly, and through that, to see and have more compassion for others and the world. When the workshop was completed, Jane and I continued our relationship through writing poetry and children's stories, attending conferences together, and going on walks. Jane and I both find a home in writing. Though I am a published writer, writing for me has been more about meditation, personal need and fulfillment, rather than as a source of income or as a profession.

In January of 2005, I asked Jane to do a poetry exchange with me. I would write a poem and email it to her' and she would write one and send it back. She said my poems to her were "communion hosts, single grapes." I felt the same about hers. When my mother died in February, and we both became busy with life, we forgot about the poem exchange until after my diagnosis in October. Then I felt inspired to ask Jane to begin writing with me again. We changed the form by speaking over the phone before and after writing. We discovered synchronicity in our writing. Our words often seemed spun on one keyboard, the ink of one pen. Each day, the muse felt the invitation and entered in.

Meanwhile, my son, Jeff, had suggested a blog, an interactive, online journal, as a way to deal with depression and isolation through cancer treatment. I, technologically challenged, had never read or even heard of one. He said it would be an easy way to stay in touch with family and friends, giving them daily, or even hourly reports. He planned to help me post, but once begun, I never stopped.

I posted, as my son Jeff, at the age of two, used to say, "by unself." Previously, my journal had been private. People ask me how I, someone so introverted, could have been so open and honest on the blog. There was nothing to hide. My doctors offered kindness, compassion, and care. I opened to receive. Throughout treatment, medical technology worked to ensure my life and the internet and email augmented my feelings of connection to the world. The blog's motto is *Carpe Moment — Seize the Moment*, and so I do.

I came to somatic work in 1992. I was in a poetry workshop with Norman Fischer at Green Gulch Zen Center in Muir Beach. Nothing was 'clicking'. Norman suggested we do some experiments with touch. We stood in a circle, and touched the shoulders of the one in front of us. We

245

then went outside to write, and when we came back inside, we read what we had written. The writing flowed together like a story written by one. It was beautiful. Norman said if we were intrigued, we should check out Charlotte Selver and her work with Sensory Awareness. I did, and that led me to understand that the journey of moving through space was as important as the destination. As I have said over and over here, the words of Charlotte carried me through. "A moment is a moment."

I also focused on the words of Elaine Chan-Scherer, who I met through email after my surgery. It is helpful to have a friend who is also awake in the night, struggling to understand the moments we are here.

I am a Rosen Method bodywork practitioner. Through Rosen, I learned to listen to my body and honor that there is a place to hold, and a place to let go. Through Rosen, through Essential Motion with Karen Roeper, and through the work of Eyes of the Beholder, I knew that when I allowed my emotions and feelings to be, they moved on through like fluffy clouds on a windy day. My intuitive energy work with Phyllis Pay and Sandra Mussey gave me tools for grounding. Each of these trainings contributed to how I experienced my illness. I practiced being in the moment, without judging what emerged. I watched myself with kind eyes.

Before I began treatment, I preferred to be the giver, the one who offered help. I think most of us do. Some say this is a characteristic of those who get breast cancer. In this year, I have learned to ask and receive. I believe the increasing number of people who have come close to death, and have been pulled through by new technology and the support of a range of therapies, will change the world, as they have learned the power of receiving these gifts that are waiting to be so generously given.

Healing still continues, though now it is more emotional than physical. I am safe enough now to release some of the layers of armor that carried me through.

In this time period, I've met a young man named Zach. He was two when I met him, and is now three. Because his mother was going through a bone marrow transplant, I was invited into his life. My work with presence continues with him. We sit and watch ladybugs, sit in clover with bees, watch crabs go in and out of holes, sit on branches inside trees. We find dead birds on the beach, even a dead seal. We visit Blackie's Pasture, and view the grave of Blackie, the horse. Sometimes Zach is sure he hears the hooves of Blackie. We have been through all the seasons together, watching the leaves change color, fall, and return. The full moon rise tells us it is time to go home. Presence with another is a gift. We can do this alone, but as Aristotle said in the Metaphysics, "The whole is more than the sum of its parts." Ask someone to share with you. It is a gift.

There is no way to thank all who have helped and guided this journey. May the knowing be enough.

LaVergne, TN USA
03 March 2010
174834LV00002B/90/P